Complexity and Healthcare

an introduction

Edited by

Kieran Sweeney

and

Frances Griffiths

Radcliffe Medical Press

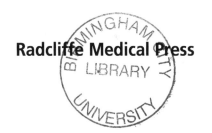

Radcliffe Medical Press Ltd
18 Marcham Road
Abingdon
Oxon OX14 1AA
United Kingdom

www.radcliffe-oxford.com
The Radcliffe Medical Press electronic catalogue and online ordering facility.
Direct sales to anywhere in the world.

British Library Cataloguing in Publication Data

A catalogue record for this book is available from the British Library.

ISBN 1 85775 559 6

Typeset by Acorn Bookwork, Salisbury, Wiltshire
Printed and bound by TJ International Ltd, Padstow, Cornwall

Contents

Foreword

'All models are wrong, some models are useful.'

This quote has been variously attributed, indicating to me that it is one of those fundamentally true insights that many people have expressed in various ways over the years. The book you hold in your hands is about 'models' – how they might be useful, and how they might be wrong.

For several centuries we have worked with the largely linear, reductionist model of science that we inherited from the likes of Descartes and Newton. This model of the way things work tells us, for example, that:

- things are best understood by taking them apart, studying the parts in depth, and then reassembling the system
- things can ultimately be 'figured out' and predicted – it is only a matter of time and the filling of current gaps in our knowledge
- there is a more-or-less linear proportionality to the world; that is, small changes will have small effects and if one desires a large effect one requires a large change.

No one can look at the tremendous advances of the last several hundred years and argue that this has not been a 'useful' model.

On the other hand, wisdom (as captured in the quote above) suggests that all models eventually reach the point where their further usefulness is seriously compromised by the degree to which they might be a bit wrong. New models are always needed to supplement the old.

In the world of science, we came to this point of compromise of the current model in the twentieth century. Heisenberg's uncertainty principle in physics, Lorentz's discovery of sensitive dependence on initial conditions in his computer models of the weather, the development of relatively simple mathematical models for chaotic phenomenon, and other advances challenge conventional notions of predictability, linearity and the pursuit of comprehensive understanding. As Bob Dylan once put it, 'The times, they are a-changing'.

Much of medicine and organisational theory is built upon the foundation of the classic scientific model. Again, let me point out that this has been extremely useful. However... could it be that we have now solved most of the problems where this model of the world is most useful? Could it be that much of the widely felt frustration in healthcare as we enter the twenty-first century is the result of the fundamental model that we bring with us no longer being so useful for many of the complex challenges we now face?

Several authors have written eloquently about the conceptual linkages between the emerging sciences of complexity and the issues of organisations in general and those of healthcare specifically. There is a relative lack, however, of practical, application-to-daily-issues advice that brings these concepts down to earth and makes them alive.

I can think of no group better stylistically equipped to step into this application gap than one composed of primary care and public health practitioners. The publication of *Complexity and Healthcare: an introduction* as a product of years of debate and practice from the Complexity in Primary Care Group, opens new paths in the largely unexplored territory of the application of complexity thinking to the daily practice of medicine and healthcare delivery. I am proud to say that I know several of the individuals in the Group and I can assure you that you will find no better guide.

I encourage you to mark a few pages in this 'field handbook', lace up your boots, adjust your backpack and get on with the journey that I firmly believe will help us deal better with our currently frustrating and complex challenges, thereby enabling us to deliver even better healthcare to the patients and the public we serve.

Paul Plsek
Consultant and author
www.directedcreativity.com
May 2002

Preface

This book has emerged from discussions held at the informal meetings of a group called the Complexity in Primary Care Group. This group came into being as a number of us in primary care in the UK were starting to read about chaos and complexity theories and to talk about them informally. We wanted to meet to learn more about them from each other and to explore whether they were of use to primary healthcare. Most of us were from general practice with a few from public health, health service management and other academic disciplines. We started to meet in late 1999 and have continued to do so three to four times a year in London. Although the authors of this book are the ones who have sat down and put the ideas on paper, many other members of the Complexity in Primary Care Group have contributed to the development of these ideas. The book would not have been written without the interaction and feedback at the meetings. The group is open to everyone who wants to participate. There is no membership fee or other payment required and no defined boundary to the group. Individuals from secondary healthcare have joined and its programme is changing as we learn more. Thus it is evolving as its members meet and interact, and in response to our environment. We hope the group is a complex adaptive system, but one with the vision to use complexity theory to improve health.

By the time you read this book the Complexity in Primary Care Group may still be meeting, it may have disbanded or developed into something else. Whatever happens to this particular group, we encourage you to discuss with your colleagues and friends, the ideas given here and so contribute to moving them forward and making them more useful to everyone – patients, carers and professionals – involved in healthcare.

At the time of publishing this book the Complexity in Primary Care Group has a website: http://www.complexityprimarycare.org which carries information about its activities.

Kieran Sweeney
Frances Griffiths
May 2002

List of contributors

Chris Burton
General Practitioner
Sanquhar Health Centre
Sanquhar, Dumfriesshire

Paul Cassidy
Clinical Governance Lead and Mental Health Lead
Gateshead PCT
General Practitioner
Teams Family Practice, Gateshead

Frances Griffiths
Senior Clinical Lecturer
University of Warwick

Alan Hassey
General Practitioner
Fisher Medical Centre (Research Unit)
Skipton, North Yorkshire

Tim Holt
General Practitioner
The Danby Practice
Danby, North Yorkshire

David Kernick
General Practitioner
Lead Researcher
St Thomas Health Centre
Exeter, Devon

Kieran Sweeney
Assistant Director, Policy and Development
Commission for Health Improvement
Lecturer in Health Services Research
Peninsula Medical School
Exeter

Barry Tennison
Assistant Director, Policy and Development
Commission for Health Improvement
Honorary Professor in Public Health and Policy
London School of Hygiene and Tropical Medicine

Introduction

Kieran Sweeney

Healthcare professionals feel challenged. Doing a job they know is important, feel is privileged, but sense is making them stressed, the challenge is complicated by a sense of paradox and confusion. Science is the currency of their discourse, sometimes the strongest weapon in their armoury, and at other times a wolf in the sheep's clothing of evidence-based medicine. We also see this paradox on a global scale. On the one hand science appears triumphant, for example with the recent publication of the genome project – 'The greatest journey ever', said *The Times*, echoing the then US President's description of the genome map as 'The most important map ever produced by man'.[1] At other times we see the Chief Medical Officer struggling to convince an increasingly sceptical public of the value of a clear and robust body of evidence supporting the safety of the mumps, measles and rubella (MMR) vaccine – all because of a weak piece of evidence suggesting a link between the vaccine and childhood autism, in a paper which had more authors on its title page than patients in the study.[2,3]

Even the National Institute for Clinical Excellence (NICE), experts at distilling vintage scientific information for the thirsty palates of the professionals, have been challenged by a sister publication, *The Drugs and Therapeutics Bulletin*, over the same body of evidence supporting the value of the new antiviral drug zanamavir in influenza.[4,5] As David Kernick reminds us in Chapter 6, research appears to have little impact on policy and organisational change, and even less on service provision.[6,7]

When asked to describe in confidence why they don't implement good evidence at times when they know it is appropriate, general practitioners give a complex answer – complex in the colloquial sense, but also, as we shall argue throughout this book, in the methodological sense too. It depends on your own personal and professional experience, doesn't it, they say; it depends on your relationship with each patient too; and, well, sometimes it's just logistically tricky, for example if you are a rural single hander.[8]

Where, one is tempted to ask, does the confusion arise? Some say that the clockwork universe of the mechanical metaphors upon which science rests is running down. Post-modernism has challenged the absoluteness of science; its directives are being challenged by relativism and the *process* of knowing.[9] And the reason science as the hegemonic model is being challenged, say others, is because the whole of healthcare has simply become more complex. While treatment of your condition will be based upon scientific evidence, your values and preferences will be factored in to the solution, and the treatment itself is likely to be delivered by a multidisciplinary team.[10]

The problem, it seems, lies with the basic explanatory model which we historically have used to manufacture, distil, interpret and disseminate scientific knowledge. Three generic problems have been identified.[9,11] In a nutshell, the conventional scientific model is resolutely reductionist, relies on a linear notion of causality, and presents itself as intellectually celibate, value-free. Let's reflect briefly on each of the elements in this triad.

Reductionism and linearity have served scientific medicine well. As practitioners in healthcare we remain to some extent disciples of Descartes, whose distinction between the mind and the body still exerts an influence over medical thinking today. Classical Newtonian mechanics served this model well, and seemed to confirm the invincibility of the notion of proportionality in cause and effect: the bigger the input, the greater the output – hence *linear* causality. Advances in optics, mathematics and technology drove our understanding of the human body as a machine deeper and deeper below the gross anatomical level, to the system level, and to the individual organ level; and in the twentieth century our medical gaze went deeper still to the cellular and ultimately the molecular level. The scientific cartographers had arrived at their destination, the ultimate ordnance survey map of the human genome. While no-one doubts the spectacular advances in medical understanding that this approach has conferred, developments outside medicine began to throw some doubt over the model's beautiful and seductive simplicity. Nature, the biologists began to tell us, appears resolutely non-linear. How, for example, do two identical cells differentiate into completely different tissues, for example nerve and skin, or bone and hair? How do they know how to do *that*? Physicists for their part were stunned when Heisenberg published his uncertainty principle. 'The foundations of physics have started moving,' Heisenberg wrote in the 1970s, 'and the motion has caused the feeling that the ground would be cut from underneath science'.[12]

Mathematicians were also gripped by non-linearity. Simple deterministic equations, if reiterated, did unpredictable things. Solutions to these simple equations got bigger, then seemed to fold over on themselves and get smaller again; the so-called Baker transformation.[13] Not much support for the conventional scientific model there. 'If things were that simple', the philosopher Derrida said, 'word would have gotten round'.

And finally, the scientific model portrayed itself as neutral and impartial, simply drawing the curtain off reality, revealing it for all to see. Think of the word '*discovery*', which implies that what was found was there all along, just waiting to be described. Yet when ordinary folk began to apply this knowledge, they didn't seem to be all that good at remaining intellectually uncontaminated. Bob Brook, explaining the reasons why British and US cardiothoracic surgeons approached identical clinical vignettes differently, appeared intellectually bankrupt: 'cultural differences' he said, 'difficult to quantify'.[14]

Five years later, a seminal paper in the *Lancet* compared prescribing practices across four European countries, all arguably using the same approach to understanding clinical science.[15] The authors found huge differences in the evidence base for the medications most frequently prescribed. In the UK, the vast majority of products were supported by good scientific research, while in France and Italy about half the most frequently prescribed medicines lacked any serious scientific basis. Something else was operating here. There were indeed other ingredients in the explanatory model's melting pot.

The recipe, some felt, lay in the paradoxes presented by considering the limitations of the present explanatory model in medicine itself. A sextet of paradoxes was proposed, and is shown in the box below. It is this sextet which brings us to the subject addressed in this book.

A sextet of paradoxes derived from the scientific model[16]

- Science appears to dominate, yet its hegemony is under threat.
- The explanatory model is linear, yet the world seems non-linear.
- The model produces evidence which is dichotomous: clinicians who use this evidence see emerging conditions whose progression remains unpredictable.
- The reductionist model denies the importance of the connectedness of its elements.
- The model is presented as value-free, yet is implemented by clinicians who are not immunised from the frailties of the human condition.
- The model does not equip the clinician for the metaphysical problems of death and dying.

This book is predicated on the notion that the current explanatory model in medicine, based ultimately on scientific positivism, is no longer sufficient *on its own* to equip the professionals working in the field to address, reflect on and understand the problems which confront them in their routine practice. Let's be quite clear what the book is *not* about. It's not about debunking science, or relegating the contribution of science in medicine to the intellectual shredder. The authors contributing to this book think that the time has come to expand the explanatory model, to seek a broader approach which addresses non-linearity, which incorporates unpredictability, and which acknowledges that no observer however dispassionate, can stand outside a system, objectively manipulating it in a precise way.

Drawing on insights from mathematics, computing, physics, systems and chaos theory, each author offers an insight into how a fresh set of metaphors from complexity can illuminate some of the seemingly intractable issues which frustrate everyday practice. Each author has written from their own professional perspective, and has been asked specifically to tell the reader about the *added* value these new (to medicine at any rate) metaphors carry for the jobbing healthcare professional. There's no point banging on about a new explanatory model just because we think the old one is flawed, we told the contributors: we have to be sure that it will confer a benefit to those who make an effort to understand it. This has been the challenge for each chapter.

The basic concepts of complexity are set out in the first chapter. Some of the terminology is strange – what exactly are attractors, what on earth is phase space, and how can the idea of emergent behaviour possibly help everyday clinicians? The introductory chapter leads the reader into this strange territory, and its author has taken great care to ensure that the journey is as transparent as possible. Chapter 2 locates this journey into complexity in the historical context. Enthusiasts who plunge into new territory like this open themselves up to the accusation of faddism, of simply seeking out the new from dissatisfaction with the old. This chapter argues that there really is nothing 'new' in challenging epistemological orthodoxy. The author paints a picture of mankind struggling with the issues which confront us today from the earliest times of recorded history.

These introductory chapters are followed by a key chapter in which the author concisely demonstrates the relevance of complexity to clinical medicine, giving examples from a range of specialties. Chapters 4 and 5 develop these links for the general practice consultation and public health respectively. In Chapter 4 Alan Hassey explains the consultation from the perspective of a complex adaptive system, and Barry Tennison, a former post-doctoral mathematician turned director of public health, applies the same approach to public health, in particular describing the relevance of non-linear mathematics to epidemiology. Chapters 5 and 6 consider the relevance of complexity to organisational thinking in healthcare. David Kernick demonstrates the value of looking at healthcare organisations at any level as complex adaptive systems. He argues that these insights might help us understand the process of change better, and explains how the notions of predictability and control are really illusory when applied to large systems. Complexity and clinical governance are discussed in Chapter 7 in a broadly similar way. At each step, the challenge is to convince the reader of the added value of thinking from the perspective of complexity. Chapter 7 demonstrates the futility of approaching clinical governance with a master plan, a 'one size fits all' solution to the emergent and unpredictable challenges of implementing clinical governance. The co-editor Frances Griffiths discusses complexity and research in Chapter 8, before offering some concluding remarks about the potential relevance of complexity to healthcare.

The reader may notice that different authors return to the same concepts, such as attractors, emergent properties and non-linearity repeatedly throughout the book. We make no apology for this, but argue that it is precisely through reading about the applicability of these ideas in different contexts that the reader will gain familiarity with the bases of these notions. The editors and the contributors are clinicians in the National Health Service, all in general practice, with the exception of our public health contributor. We have all struggled with the notions of complexity, have developed a basic familiarity with them, and present our own insights to help the reader to understand them too. We all hope that your new understanding of complexity will kindle your enthusiasm to dig deeper.

References

1   *The Times*, June 23, 2000.

2   Elliman D and Bedford H (2001) MMR vaccine: the continuing saga. *BMJ*. **322**: 183–4.

3   Wakefield AJ, Murch SH, Anthony A *et al.* (1998) Ileal lymphoid nodular hyperplasia, non-specific colitis and pervasive developmental disorder in children. *Lancet*. **351**: 637–41.

4   National Institute for Clinical Excellence (2000) *Guidance on the Use of Zanamivir in the Treatment of Influenza*. Technology Appraisal Guidance No 15, November. National Institute for Clinical Excellence, London.

5   Editorial (2001) Why not Zanamivir? *Drugs and Therapeutics Bulletin*. **39(2)**: 9–10.

6   Black N (2001) Evidence based policy: proceed with care. *BMJ*. **323**: 275–9.

7   Sheldon T (2001) It ain't what you do but the way that you do it. *Journal of Health Services Research and Policy*. **6**: 3–5.

8   Freeman A and Sweeney K (2001) Why general practitioners do not implement evidence. *BMJ*. **323**: 1100–3.

9   Kernick D and Sweeney K (2001) Post normal medicine. *Family Practice*. **18**: 356–8.

10   Plsek P and Greenhalgh T (2001) The challenge of complexity in health care. *BMJ.* **323**: 625–8.

11   Dixon M and Sweeney K (2000) *The Human Effect in Medicine*. Radcliffe Medical Press, Oxford.

12   Heisenberg W (1971) *Physics and Beyond*. Harper & Row, New York.

13   Capra F (1996) *The Web of Life*. Bantam, Doubleday Dell Publishing, New York.

14   Brook RH, Park RE, Winslow CM *et al.* (1988) Diagnosis and treatment of coronary disease: a comparison of doctors' attitudes in the USA and the UK. *Lancet.* **189**: 7550—3.

15   Garratini S and Garratini L (1993) Pharmaceutical prescribing in four European countries. *Lancet.* **342**: 1191–2.

16   Sweeney K and Kernick D (2002) Clinical evaluation: constructing a new model for post normal medicine. *Journal of Clinical Evaluation*. In press.

CHAPTER ONE

Introduction to complexity

Chris Burton

The central idea of this book, that complexity and the study of complex adaptive systems are a valuable way of looking at health-care, is new. The science behind complexity is still being explored and much of its vocabulary is unfamiliar. As old words ('complexity', 'chaos', 'emergence') have acquired new or specific meanings, it is important to set the scene for subsequent chapters by introducing the concepts behind complexity. In some cases familiar words will be used to mean specific things – for example 'chaos' describes something that looks random, but in fact has an underlying cause and structure. In other cases new and intimidating phrases such as 'self-organising criticality' will be invoked to describe things which can be readily understood, although not easily encapsulated in a few words.

Complexity as we describe it is certainly not cut and dried, nor are there theories which can be proved – at least not in a conventional scientific way. However, there are elements within it which can be consistently and predictably demonstrated. Furthermore, complexity offers new insights into many aspects of our daily work so that to some extent we end up resorting to the aphorism that if it looks like complexity and behaves like complexity, then probably it is complexity.

At the heart of complexity there is a set of key features.

Box 1.1 Key features of a complex system

- Complex systems consist of multiple components. Such systems are understood by observing the rich interaction of these components, not simply understanding the system's structure.
- The interaction between components can produce unpredictable behaviour.
- Complex systems have a history and are sensitive to initial conditions.
- Complex systems interact with and are influenced by their environment.
- The interactions between elements of the system are non-linear, that is to say that the result of any action depends on the state of the elements at the time as well as the size of the input. Small inputs may have large effects, and vice versa.
- The interactions generate new properties, called 'emergent behaviours' of the system, which cannot be explained through studying the elements of the system however much detail is known.
- In complex systems such emergent behaviour cannot be predicted.
- Complex systems are open systems: when observed, the observer becomes part of the system.

The aim of this introductory chapter is to explain the terms in use, and how people use them to get to the ideas at the heart of complexity. In the first section, *mathematics in an unpredictable world*, we see how ideas which began in the rarified world of mathematics can be useful in understanding complexity as we meet it in the real world. This section touches on the phenomenon of deterministic chaos and the notion of attractors.

The second section, *biology meets computers*, looks at developments such as neural networks and artificial life simulations which offer new insights into the way natural systems develop and covers ideas such as emergence, fitness, landscapes and rules. As well as having a relevance for biomedical systems, many of the principles appear applicable to anything that can evolve, grow and decay, be it a cell, an organism or an organisation.

The third section, *joining things together*, draws out the ways that connections, non-linear interactions and emergent phenomena generate order and strength within complex systems.

Mathematics in an unpredictable world

Thinking in spaces

In healthcare, we tend to think of conditions as discrete entities. Conventional medical knowledge tells us that there are distinct illnesses which are either present or not, and that these illnesses can be clearly described and are separable with clear boundaries. In reality, some cases of illness are very clear, such as a classic pneumonia, but other cases do not quite match the classic descriptions. Illnesses also have many features which extend beyond the dis-ease of a particular organ. Pain, fear, anxiety and depression can all accompany a serious illness episode. Personal, family and social factors are involved too. The illness experience has multiple dimensions. Mathematics can help us understand both the idea of categories without clear boundaries and the idea of multiple dimensions.

As a way of addressing the notion of multiple dimensions, mathematics developed the idea of spaces, in which all potential values for something can be found. It is easiest to start with numbers. For instance in primary school we learn about whole numbers. Later we realise that there are many more, for example 2.674 and 5.789421, although often we round up or down to the nearest whole number to get something that is 'good enough' and easier to handle. If you think of all possible numbers – at least those up to five decimal places – between 0 and 10 as occupying a line, then there will be ten whole numbers amongst the 100 000 numbers comprising this particular number space.

This example has only one dimension and it is something we can all visualise easily. It can be made a little more complex by moving up to two dimensions, which gives us a way of plotting coordinates on a map, or even three dimensions, which allows us to plot a position within a cube. In medicine, things rarely have just three dimensions. Think how many different ways there are of categorising a pain, or the interaction of two people. As described by mathematics, these 'phase spaces' need not be restricted to three or four dimensions; the number of dimensions reflects the characteristics of the system itself.

As a way of visualising six-dimensional space and the possibilities within it, consider all possible sequences of exactly six letters. That gives 26^6 or just over 300 million possibilities. Within this six-letter word space will be all the six-letter words in the English language (actually any language, but we'll ignore the others for now). There will also be a much larger number of non-words as well as words that used to exist but don't anymore, and some which have not yet come into existence. For instance, putnox is not yet a term of abuse but might one day become so. When one considers the distribution of words in this space it is clear that the words, whilst at a first glance appearing to be randomly distributed, are not. There are clusters of words close together: cattle, candle, cantor all sit close to each other in some dimensions whilst not in others, as do words ending in -s or -es or -ing. There are also great tracts of this six-letter space in which no words exist and all the entries are, for now, non-words, for example those beginning xw- or xz. If you have got this far, you have demonstrated that, by turning a blind eye to some of the detail and by selectively viewing a few of the dimensions at a time, the human brain can think of distributions in multiple dimensions. Similarly, in healthcare we can think of illness as having multiple dimensions, although we may only consider a few of the dimensions at a time.

Using the idea of multidimensional phase space can help us understand categories of disease without clear boundaries. Instead of thinking of a person's illness as a walled off and separate pigeon hole, it can be useful to think of it as a point within a multidimensional illness space. If we take pain as an example of a symptom of illness, we can identify at least six dimensions to the pain (Box 1.2). In terms of the pain it causes, the illness can be plotted on all these dimensions. There will be other dimensions too as well as those related to the pain. If many individuals' illnesses were plotted in illness phase space there would be clusters of points which we would recognise as illnesses, such as pneumonia or heart attack. There would be points near the centre of the cluster 'classic illness'

Box 1.2 Six possible dimensions for the symptom pain

- Location
- Radiation
- Duration
- Nature
- Intensity
- Associated disturbance

---

and other points towards the edge of the cluster: there would be no distinct boundary to the cluster.

Attractors in space

Stay with the idea of multidimensional phase space and an illness as a point plotted in this space. We can take an example such as 'sore throat space' and plot two of its dimensions on a chart (Figure 1.1). One axis is local severity of pain and the other is systemic upset. Any sore throat can be represented by a position on this chart.

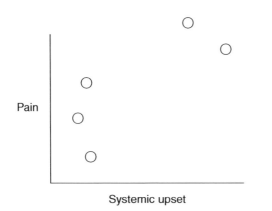

Figure 1.1 Sore throat space with five different points.

If, for episodes of sore throat, we make several measurements of these two values over a period of time, say several days, then a trajectory for sore throat can be drawn. Figure 1.2 uses the points from Figure 1.1 to demonstrate the trajectories of two episodes, one bacterial and the other viral. Although setting off into different areas of sore throat space, both coincide on the recovery pathway. If many sore throats were plotted on this chart they would all follow slightly different trajectories but most of them would follow a route somewhere near the bacterial trajectory or the viral trajectory as shown in Figure 1.2. There would be two channels on the chart along which most cases would move. These channels, or regions of space, where the trajectories are fairly close are called attractors.

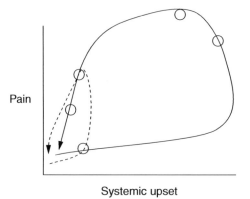

Figure 1.2 Trajectories through sore throat space over time, bacterial (solid line) and viral (dotted line) infections.

An attractor is the area that a system moves towards and where it will tend to stay. Consider a perfectly curved bowl with a marble in it. However you move the marble it will always end up at the bottom of the bowl. The bottom of the bowl is an attractor. Attractors are not always a single point. Consider a swinging pendulum where the system settles towards a pattern of movement which is repeated. The attractor is the shape traced out by the pendulum over time. These two examples are very simple attractors. More complex attractors are considered later in this chapter.

Let us return to clinical practice to consider hidden attractors. Figure 1.3 shows an imaginary consultation time-quality space for GP consultations. It shows the broad association between consultation length and quality. Figure 1.4 shows a similar space with the trajectory of a series of consultations from one surgery. For the same surgery, Figure 1.5 shows a mapping in consultation space comparing quality with a new variable 'lateness' which is a property not of the current consultation length but of the sum of the length of all previous consultations. This way of looking at the data shows four points (filled circles) fairly close together on the left of the chart, with three of them occurring in sequence. These correspond to the four similar data points (filled circles) in Figure 1.4 whose relationship is a little less clear as the consultations themselves are of widely varying length, albeit of poorer quality. The redrawing of consultation space using the dimension of lateness rather than consultation length has highlighted a different attractor, 'running late, poor quality', which is not immediately obvious from the original data. It was there all along, it just wasn't obvious until we looked in the right way. By looking at the data differently we have uncovered a hidden attractor. The concept of attractors, which is central to complex systems, will be explored further in subsequent chapters in the book.

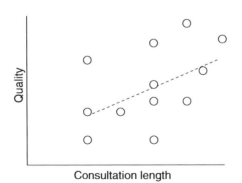

Figure 1.3 Consultation space for GP consultations, showing the association between consultation length and quality.

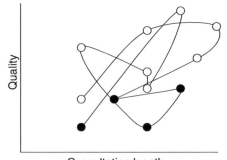

Figure 1.4 Trajectory through consultation space for a series of consultations during a GP surgery.

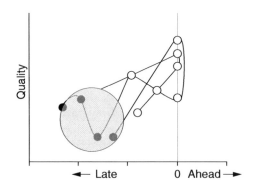

Figure 1.5 Trajectory through a transformed consultation space, greyed area represents a 'running late – poor quality' attractor.

Non-linearity

A simple example of a non-linear interaction is familiar to anyone who has experienced a demanding toddler in a supermarket:

> 'I want a sweetie' – quiet request.
> 'Not just now dear' – gentle refusal.
> 'I Want a sweetie' – firmer request.
> 'Not just now dear' – identical refusal.
> 'I Want A Sweetie' – strong request.
> 'I said "No" ' – strong refusal.
> 'I WANT A SWEETIE' – very strong request.

Now, what comes next? It could either be:
   'All right then' – capitulation, or
   'I SAID "NO"' – an even stronger refusal.

The way that the mother and toddler interacted in the same encounter the previous week, and in different encounters earlier today, and how they both interacted with lots of other people over the previous few hours will all influence how the interaction works out. However, the bottom line is that at any time, whilst the potential outcomes from an incremental rise in the request can be described, the actual one which occurs cannot be predicted in advance. This simple illustration demonstrates some of the key principles of complex systems, outlined in Box 1.1. The system (in this case the interaction of mother and daughter) has a history, it is sensitive to initial conditions, and its future cannot be precisely predicted, either in time or in direction.

A mathematical example of a non-linear interaction in a complex system is an equation developed to understand how a population with limited resources, for example fish in a pond, waxes and wanes over time. As a rule, the larger the population of fish grows, the more likely it is to 'outstretch' its resources, and the smaller it is, the better opportunity it has of growing back. The force driving its growth is the same throughout and is represented by a constant k. The population density at any time is represented by x (a value between 0 and 1, where 1 represents complete saturation of the environment). Using these criteria $(1-x)$ is equivalent to the available space within the environment.

The growth formula which describes how this kind of ecosystem waxes and wanes is k multiplied by x multiplied by $(1-x)$ as follows:

$$x_1 = kx(1-x)$$

The result x_1 of this equation is then fed in as x in the next iteration of the equation which is repeated many times building up a series of results representing the population over time. If the growth force constant k is too low (below 3 in this model) the population dies out quickly. However, if k is between 3 and 3.5 and the equation is repeated many times, then strange things begin to happen. Instead of linear or smoothly cycling growth, the value of x begins to vary unpredictably. Sometimes there will be almost no change and then a series of widely swinging results. These apparently bizarre results are not due to error creeping in and are completely reproducible by running precisely the same equation again with the same values. (However, if the starting values or the value of k are only fractionally different, the results of the equation will be completely different.)

This pattern of apparently unpredictable change determined by a non-linear equation is termed 'deterministic chaos' (often shortened to 'chaos'). A relatively simple numerical system can generate immensely complicated numerical outcomes through repeated non-linear interaction. Systems manifesting this characteristic are termed 'chaotic systems'.

Chaos

Chaotic systems demonstrate features which are useful in understanding complexity, and in particular attractors and fractal scaling.

Simple attractors have been described earlier but chaotic systems have a novel kind of attractor. Whilst chaotic systems are reproducible, one of their key features is that they never quite repeat themselves. Often they can appear to lock on to an almost regular pattern, and then after a while drift away from it. Analysis of the trajectory may demonstrate an attractor towards which the system tends to move, which is neither a single point nor a repeated loop. These are called 'strange attractors' because when plotted out they reveal not simple geometric patterns but complex, although clearly ordered, shapes. Strange attractors are a typical feature of chaotic systems. A physical model that can help us understand this is the executive desk toy of a pendulum suspended between two or three magnets. The swing will constantly change around the attractors of the magnets. Although such a system obeys a fairly straightforward set of equations, these are dependent on the position at the start and the exact strength of magnetic field. As it is impossible to reproduce these conditions exactly, it is not possible to predict precisely where, or in what direction, the pendulum will be swinging in, for example a dozen swings, although we know it will be swinging somewhere between the magnets which are its attractors. The margins of the attractors are the boundaries of the system, but we cannot know precisely where, within the attractors' boundaries, the system will be at any one moment in time.

The limitation of chaos, as described here, is that it is a system that is running independently of its environment. For instance, the fish in a pond scenario assumes there is a constant supply of food with no change, and no sudden arrival of a party of anglers. Whilst it seems increasingly clear that many biological systems run on a non-linear basis, few are sufficiently isolated from their environment for chaos to be easily demonstrated. A powerful exception is heart rate variability, which whilst susceptible to environmental change has a limited number of possibilities (go faster, go slower). Other patterns very strongly suggestive of chaos can be seen but, in general, biological and organisational systems interact with their environment in multiple ways so that underlying patterns are diluted, or dissipated by the environment. However, the principle of non-linear interaction, whose pattern creates its hidden attractors, is fundamental to complex systems. The key difference between chaos and a complex system is that the complex system is constantly adapting to, and co-evolving with, its environment.

These ideas of non-linear dynamic systems, containing strange attractors and non-linear interaction, and interacting with the environment, offer exciting metaphors for studying healthcare and are explored further in later chapters.

Biology meets computers

Complexity does not just depend on numerical manipulation but on insights drawn from more observational sciences. Although naturalists have meticulously recorded many kinds of biological data, it is only with the advent of modern computers that experiments involving simulations have been possible. Simulations, whilst clearly artificial, are currently the best way for observing systems which in themselves are unmeasurable (involving too many things, or taking too long) but which defy reductionist analysis. This section will describe simulated models of evolution, behaviour and life itself to examine how complex systems interact.

Evolution and co-evolution

This next section discusses evolution broadly in biological terms, and will refer to fitness (as in Darwin's survival of the fittest) to mean ability to flourish in the environment. It could also be read in social terms to refer to effectiveness of members of an organisation, or of a monetary economy where change can either work for (increase fitness) or against (decrease fitness) them.

The story of evolution, as simplistically taught, seems to be one of relentless progress and improvement. Genes change bit by bit, the best changes win out and so the best genes inexorably survive. Furthermore, there is an implicit assumption that any change, if beneficial in the short term, is part of a progression up an evolutionary ladder.

However, real life evolution happens in ecosystems with multiple components and it may be that what is best for one organism depends on what is best for others around it. No organism evolves without changing its environment in some way. At a simple level imagine a world of herbivores in which a new creature evolves the capacity to hunt down and eat other animals. For a while its evolution gives it great potential – lots of food and no competition. However, before long, the herbivores become so scarce that the carnivores can no longer sustain themselves, not least because the remaining herbivores are completely hidden by the burgeoning undergrowth. If on the other hand the herbivores evolve strategies for hiding or running away, the balance is restored, at least until the next steps in the evolutionary process. Evolution depends on co-evolution.

Theoretical models using computer simulations of populations, gradual change and mutual interdependency provide a number of interesting scenarios.

● In situations where each entity (be it a gene or an organism) is dependent on few other entities, then an evolutionary change will have a clearly beneficial or harmful effect on its fitness. For example, a colony of bacteria on an agar plate that evolved a way of multiplying more quickly would have an advantage; the faster the multiplication, the greater the advantage.

- In situations where each entity is directly dependent on very many other entities in the system, – and remember this is a reciprocal arrangement – then improving the fitness of one entity produces widespread diminution of the fitness of other components, which in turn affects the one that originally changed and so on. The net result is that the average fitness of the entities in the system remains the same, but fitness is continuously redistributed in an unpredictable way.
- Somewhere in between lies an optimum pattern with moderate numbers of direct interdependencies. Here, evolutionary changes by an individual to increase its own fitness increase the average fitness of all the entities in the system.

This last point is worth restating. We are used to interaction between entities in a system leading to one gaining fitness at another's expense (in terms of both biological systems and human organisations or economies). The overall fitness (common good or capital, if you want to view this socially or economically) doesn't change, it is just redistributed. Here we have the interaction increasing not just the fitness of one part of the system, but adding new fitness to the system.

Neurophysiology

Biology is not all about clever simulations. Laboratory research is also yielding insights into complexity. Neurophysiology offers insights into the nature of complex systems.

At the level of the single nerve cell, the neurone, it is clear that here is a biological system run on non-linear principles. As anyone who did a first year physiology course may remember, neurones receive chemical messages from the synapses with adjacent cells. Until a critical level is reached the neurone does nothing. Once that level is reached the neurone fires, and an electrical impulse travels along the cell to release neurotransmitters to pass the signal to the next neurones in the chain. Thereafter for a brief refractory period, no matter how hard the cell is stimulated, it will not fire until it is ready.

A feature of nerve cells that has been hypothesised for many years but is only now becoming demonstrable, is that nerves and their connections, at least in areas where learning is taking place, are steadily changing. There is increasing evidence to suggest, for instance, that the more a connection between two neurones is used, the stronger it becomes. As the connection gets stronger, it takes less and less of a stimulus to fire the neurone. In this way a well-used path for transmission of an impulse becomes progressively easier to trigger. This effect may explain phenomena such as learning, but also casts light on some of the problems of chronic pain, where prolonged stimulation of neural pain pathways may heighten sensitivity to pain even when the original cause has been removed.

At this level of interconnected nerve cells, we see another characteristic of complex systems, their sensitivity to their history. Chronic pain can be regarded as a non-linear system with a history, for the effect of stimulating the nerve depends not just on the last few milliseconds, but on the last few days, or months or years of its interactions.

Neurophysiology is moving beyond the study of a single cell to more complex networks of cells. These can now be studied either in cultured networks of neurones or in computer simulations of nerves and their connections known as neural networks. Neural networks have contributed to our understanding of several features of complexity. One particular aspect is the idea of distributed knowledge.

We tend to think of the brain storing information in particular places, for example a different area in which memories of other people's faces are stored; one cell, or group of cells for each person's face that we have known. Work on neural networks suggests that this type of representational memory may not be correct. Simulated networks, can be taught to recognise patterns, for example visual or sound patterns. The network 'learns' by repeatedly adjusting the balance between neurones by transmitting a certain signal.

In networks such as these, which are capable of learning to recognise something external, there is no representation of each object within the system. Instead the *pattern of connections* holds the memory. The knowledge is distributed through the network in the connections rather than each piece of knowledge being stored, or represented, in one place. Remove a few neurones and the results of remembering may not be quite so good, but they will largely remain. Similarly with the brain; if we forget someone's name, we can usually remember it later; it is not permanently lost. Distributed knowledge is a valuable feature of complex networks, and demonstrates the key feature of such systems: the behaviour of the system results from rich interaction of the constituent parts. In addition, a reductionist approach to analysing such a system which would deconstruct the brain into axons, myelin sheaths and nerve cells, would simply fail to tell us how it behaved.

Rules and behaviour

Watch a flock of birds in the sky and it appears as if some unseen hand is guiding them. Each bird seems to know where to go as if some communication system was telling them. But what if such behaviour is actually the manifestation of some simple rules? From this conjecture, and largely by trial and error rather than hypothetical deduction from real observations, computer scientists developed a set of three rules which, when applied to a flock of simulated birds, produced realistic behaviour. The rules of this simulation are described and discussed further in Chapter 7. The idea that local interactions following simple rules can lead to the emergence of apparently complex behaviours of the whole group is fundamental to the study of complex systems. This highlights the importance of all the individual agents in a system. The system develops according to the way its members interact with each other and their environment.

The ideas of simple rules and emergent properties are in many ways a mirror image of the concept of attractors. On one hand the rules specify the emergent behaviour, on the other the behaviour is analysed to identify fundamental attractors. Whether complex human systems can be modelled with simple rules is debatable but, particularly in the field of management, much effort is going into attempts to identify and modify rules, or their mirror images, attractors. These attempts are discussed further in the chapters on healthcare organisations and clinical governance later in the book.

Joining things together

Emerging order

The modelling of mutual interdependency producing emergent properties we have just seen, which, in evolutionary terms, increases the survival advantage rather than just redistributing it, is potentially very exciting. Such appearances of order out of apparently disordered activity can also be seen in a number of other areas.

Imagine a heap of sand on a table and the effect of adding more sand, one grain at a time to the top of the heap. In reality, this is a simple physical system which, despite appearing random, has a remarkable order to it. For a while the heap grows and then landslides start. They can be small trickles, or major collapses; they are unpredictable in their size and their timing yet each is provoked by the same trigger, a falling grain of sand. However, measuring the size of these landslides reveals a consistent pattern which suggests they are not simply random. The frequency of landslides is inversely related to the size. This relationship is logarithmic rather than linear – if the smallest landslide is of two grains and happens once for every n grains dropped, a grain landslide twice as big will happen every n^2 grains and a landslide 10 times bigger every n^{10}.

This heap of inert sand is throwing off apparently random patterns of landslides, although behind them is a clear physical relationship governing their size and frequency. This pattern has been termed 'self-organising criticality'. There is a form of order, arising from within a system which appears disordered. This is a little like the description of deterministic chaos, whereby small changes can produce marked transformations in a system which has strong but often invisible attractors embedded within it.

A computer simulation that demonstrates order arising out of apparent disorder comprises a grid of squares like a giant chess board. It has a set of simple rules (such as, if the square adjacent to you changes colour then ...) and a single change can be transmitted across the grid in patterns that appear random and then suddenly show remarkable order. In these systems there appear to be three general areas within the system space. First, there are stable states, when change tends to be slow, linear and incremental. Second, there are chaotic states, in which the system goes through unpredictable and apparently random changes. Change certainly happens here, but so quickly and unpredictably that it can rarely be harnessed. Third, and most interestingly, is the area where the emergence of order and self-organisation takes place. This seems to be at the interface between the slow changing stable states and the rapidly changing uncontrollable areas of chaos. This area has been termed 'the edge of chaos' and appears to be the cutting edge, the peak of the wave, the place where the biggest gains are to be made – a thrilling and challenging place to be.

Conclusion

This chapter has described the key features of complex systems to provide a basis for understanding the ideas explored in the rest of the book. It has also demonstrated the *additional* value of using the metaphors from complexity to help us understand many familiar complex systems which we encounter in real life, including our daily healthcare practice. Multidimensional phase space may initially seem a curious notion, but it does help us observe illness experiences, and begins to explain why the same illness, for example heart failure, can appear to progress quite differently in different people. Attractors help us understand why complex systems can remain around the same approximate area of phase space for prolonged periods. This notion will be explored further in the context of clinical governance, when the term is applied to the nature of clinical governance in a particular locality. The example of distributed knowledge shows us how it is through the rich interaction of agents that the pattern of behaviour of a system emerges. In an era in which medicine increasingly doubts the value of reductionism, the time is ripe for exploring the additional benefits derived from the insights of complexity theory.

Further reading

Cilliers P (1998) *Complexity and Postmodernism*. Routledge, London. Despite the daunting title, this is a remarkably clear book which introduces complexity to the general reader, particularly from the social science perspective.

Cohen J and Stewart I (1994) *The Collapse of Chaos: discovering simplicity in a complex world*. Penguin, London. This book introduces complexity, particularly from the biological perspective.

Gleick J (1997) *Chaos*. Minerva, London. The original lay reader's guide to chaos theory, readable on a train. The author captures the excitement in the early discoveries of non-linearity.

Kauffman S (1995) *At Home in the Universe: the search for laws of complexity*. Penguin, London. This book explores, and draws together, threads of complexity from many different perspectives and disciplines.

Plsek P and Greenhalgh T (2001) Complexity science: the challenge of complexity in health care. *BMJ*. **323**: 625–8. The first in a series of four articles introducing complexity in healthcare.

Stacey R (2000) *Strategic Management and Organisational Dynamics: the challenge of complexity*. Pearson Education, London. One of the best introductions to complexity in organisations and management.

Stewart I (1997) *Does God Play Dice: the new mathematics of chaos*. Penguin, London. Invaluable descriptions of non-linearity and chaos although not much on complexity.

Zimmerman BJ, Lindberg C and Plsek P (1998/2001) *Edgeware: insights from complexity science for health care leaders*. VHA, Texas. Much of the content of this is available online at the website of the Plexus Institute, an independent and increasingly influential group of healthcare advisers and complexity thinkers based in the USA. http://www.plexusinstitute.com/edgeware/archive/index.html

CHAPTER TWO

History of complexity

Kieran Sweeney

Summary

Complexity seems exciting. It has the huge appeal of offering fresh potential for understanding systems, whether these 'systems' are patients, consultations, public health, organisations such as PCTs, or the whole NHS. But is our current interest in the topic justified? Is it just a way of challenging received wisdom, an irresponsible distraction for researchers who have grown tired of conventional explanatory models? Or, in exploring this challenging and rapidly evolving field, are we forming part of a long tradition of enquiry into the nature of knowledge, of how we understand reality, of how we make sense of the world and our place in it? In this chapter I try to place our interest in complexity in a historical tradition of enquiry going back to the dawn of Western thought. In quoting from Pythagoras, Aristotle, Epicurus and Heraclitus, I try to show how these, the earliest philosophers in Western civilisation, struggled with the same profound issues of reality and with how to understand it. In citing Descartes, Bacon and Koch I make the point that as healthcare professionals we are enacting a philosophical tradition, however subconsciously – in our case, we are disciples of Descartes. And by drawing on examples from art, poetry and music, I argue that the debate is a universal one, exploring the fundamental nature of explanation, representation and interpretation of knowledge. The interest in complexity is not mere faddism. In pursuing the insights of complexity and exploring how it might apply to healthcare, we are merely foot soldiers in a long tradition, standing on the shoulders of giants.

Introduction

When a movement as new, radical, and challenging as complexity descends upon an inherently conservative profession such as medicine, champions of the new movement expose themselves to the accusation of faddism. This is an accusation that we have to address head on. As health professionals expressing an interest in complexity, are we simply dabbling in a new and exciting area of knowledge, which allows us irresponsibly to challenge long-cherished conventions, or are we part of something that is more fundamental? In supporting the latter view, we focus on two key notions about the nature of systems which are central to this book. These are the tension between the *structure* of a system and the *pattern* created by the interaction of its components, and the tension between *determinism* and *unpredictability* in systems. How certain can we be of how and where a system will move to through time? Here we use the word 'system' generically, to indicate a perceived whole whose components interact richly because they continually affect each other and operate towards a common sense of purpose.[1] In this chapter I argue that these two notions – structure versus pattern, determinism versus unpredictability have been debated for almost as long as knowledge has been recorded as a central feature of man's struggle to understand nature.

Graeco-Roman origins

At the dawn of Western thought, references to the relationship between the structure of matter and its pattern or form can be found in the writings of the earliest philosophers. The study of substance can be traced back to the work of Thales and Parmenides. They asked, 'What is reality made of?' and 'What are the basic building blocks of matter?' The first answers from the Greek philosophers to these questions identified the four fundamental elements of earth, air, fire and water. These, the Greeks said, were the fundamental constituents of matter. Theirs was the first recorded dialogue in Western thought about how to understand the fundamental substances which constituted reality. The debate continues today and can be traced, for example, in biology. The earliest taxonomies in biology were at the level of species, at that time the most fundamental level of order known to that discipline. In the late eighteenth and nineteenth centuries, particularly with the advances in optics, classification at the level of organisms was introduced, and then with the discovery of cells and cellular components the reduction to constituent parts went deeper and deeper. But the questions were still the same: what are the building blocks of matter and what is reality made of?

Running in parallel with this debate throughout history has been a similar enquiry into the study of form or pattern. This can be traced back to Pythagoras. In his writings, we recognise the first stated distinction between structure or matter and pattern or form.[2] Aristotle also recognised the distinction between matter and form, arguing that matter contained the essence of all things but only as a potentiality. Form or pattern was what gave this essence actuality.

The Greeks also struggled with the notion of determinism. Is the universe ruled by deterministic laws? Are we able to predict what will happen to systems precisely, and if so how? These questions were debated in the pre-Socratic era at the very start of Western rational thought. Epicurus, a follower of Democritus, supported the conventional belief at that time, namely that the world was made up of atoms and a void. The atoms, the Greeks considered at that time, fell through the void at the same speed and on parallel paths. This model immediately posed the problem of how to explain novelty, and it also raised the problem of human freedom: what could be the meaning of human freedom if the world was deterministically composed of atoms in this way? Epicurus proposed a solution which he termed 'clinamen'. Lucretius described Epicurus' solution thus, 'While the first bodies are being carried downwards by their own weight in straight lines through the void, at times quite uncertain and at uncertain places, they deviate slightly from their course, just enough to have been defined as having changed direction'.[3] In an era struggling with the discomfort of Heisenberg's uncertainty principle, that description written thousands of years ago seems strangely contemporary. Heraclitus, contributing to the same debate, argued that novelty need not be introduced, if the nature of *becoming* was stressed. Popper records Heraclitus as arguing that 'truth lies in having grasped the essential becoming of nature, that is having represented it as implicitly infinite, as a process in itself'.[4] For his part, Plato linked truth with being, arguing in favour of the unchanging reality which was beyond becoming. However, recognising that this position debased life, the human predicament, and the freedom to think, Plato concludes in *The Sophist* that we needed both being and becoming.[5] This duality has tested Western philosophy ever since.

The influence of Descartes

The contemporary accepted thinking upon which the practice of medicine is based derives from the work of the seventeenth century philosopher and mathematician Rene Descartes. He introduced the notion of dualism, which has shaped thinking about clinical medicine ever since. On one side, Descartes argued, is matter, *res extensa*, which could be described by geometry and on the other, the mind, *res cogitans*[6]. Descartes' expression of mind/body dualism and his development of the ontological concept of disease, brought rational positivist thinking to the centre of medicine in a way which remains virtually unaltered at the start of the twenty-first century. Bacon's influence around this time was substantial too. He first related the manifestations of illness in real life to the pathological changes in the morbid state in his classic *Advancement of Learning*.

The conceptual framework laid out by Descartes, in whose work the dominant metaphor for the body is the machine, was hugely supported by the development by Isaac Newton of classical (Newtonian) mechanics. Newton's mechanical series of laws provided a highly desirable and suitably mechanistic set of metaphors for medical practice to use. One of the earliest examples of the application of Newtonian mechanics in clinical practice was Harvey's description of the circulation in 1628. Harvey was the first to describe the notion of circulation as the basis for the movement of blood – previous explanatory models were based on a poorly developed notion of ebb and flow. Harvey based his explanation on the simple but, at the time, quite radical observation that the amount of blood which flowed from the heart in an hour far exceeded the total blood volume. Harvey's contribution is still considered to be the basis of physiology today and is utterly central to the rationalist basis of clinical medical practice.[7-10]

The nineteenth and twentieth centuries

It was really in the last two centuries that a rationalist, positivist and reductionist approach to scientific thinking in medicine became firmly entrenched. The nineteenth century saw the dawn of hospital medicine in Paris. Foucault identifies Bichat, a Parisienne anatomist, as a key influence. 'The greatest break-through in the history of Western medicine', Foucault observes, 'dates precisely from the moment clinical experience became the anatomo-clinical gaze'.[11]

Advances in technology, particularly in optics, supported the development of germ theory, which gained its first major triumph in 1891 with the publication of Koch's postulates. Koch proposed that a disease could be defined as the combination of three elements, the causal agent, the pathological lesion and the clinical syndrome.[10] Further developed by Pasteur, Koch's postulates set the scene for the development of germ theory as a central component in the practice of medicine in the Western world.

The influence of romanticism

The dominance of Cartesian dualism and its reductionist approach to thinking throughout the seventeenth century and subsequently did not go completely unchallenged. The romantic poets offered the first strong opposition. Put most succinctly by William Blake, the mystical poet and writer, the romantic position was summarised as follows:

'May God us keep
From single vision and Newton's sleep.'

The romantic view was perhaps more eloquently expressed by Wordsworth in *The Tables Turned*:

> Our meddling instinct mis-shapes the beauteous form of
>   things
> We murder to dissect.
>
> (lines 26–28[12])

In the twentieth century these poetic notions were developed by TS Eliott, among others. His poem *The Rock*, first published in 1934, eloquently describes wisdom as what complexity theorists would call an emergent property, arising out of the interaction of sub-components of information:

> Where is the life we have lost in loving?
> Where is the wisdom we have lost in knowledge?
> Where is the knowledge we have lost in information?

In Germany, poets and philosophers in the romantic movement revisited the Aristotelian tradition, focusing their reflections on organic form. It was Goethe, the dominant figure among the German romanticists, who first introduced the term morphology to indicate his predilection for studying biology from a dynamic and developmental point of view. 'Each creature', wrote Goethe, 'is but a patterned gradation of one great harmonious whole'.[13]

The understanding of organic form, of the pattern produced by the interaction of components, was an important feature of the philosophy of Immanuel Kant. Kant felt that dogmatic rationalism was too constraining to describe the human predicament. He faced up to the conflict between this notion of human freedom and the scientific method developed by Galileo, Bacon and others. In his three critiques of the scope of human reason, action and judgement, Kant proposed a new paradigm of nature which attempted to resolve the contradictions or 'antinomies' presented by the positivists. Kant distinguished between mechanisms and organisms. The former were subject to linear cause and effect links. This kind of linear causality predominated in science and accounted for both stability and change in a way that was entirely predictable. Organisms, however, Kant argued, were to be understood in a systemic way. Here, causality was predominantly formative, in that it was in the self-organising interaction of the parts, that those parts and subsequently the whole emerged.[14] Science, Kant argued, could only offer mechanical explanations but it was clear that there were areas where such explanations were inadequate and needed to be supplemented by considering nature as in some ways purposeful.[15] In his description of organisms, which Kant contrasted with machines, he makes a crucial distinction which would not be unfamiliar today to those interested in complex theory. In machines, Kant argued, parts exist for each other, whereas in organisms they also exist *by means of* each other in the sense of producing one another.[16] 'We must think of each part as an organ', Kant wrote, 'that produces the other parts, so that each reciprocally produces the other ... because of this the organism will be both an organised and self-organising being'.[17]

The role of Darwin

Darwin's two major works *The Origin of Species* (1859) and *The Descent of Man* (1871) places him centrally in the historical picture describing the thinking on stability, change, pattern and form. In the hope that this brief summary does not do a disservice to Darwin's profound and challenging views, the main theme of both his major books concerned an organism's survival in its local environment. More than anything else, Darwin argued, the organism's body parts served this particular function of survival. The same struggle can be seen at species level, where the individual organisms can be considered the equivalent of the body parts of the single individual. Species, Darwin argued, are altered by variations among the individual organisms, some of which are beneficial, enhance survival and thus favour continued reproduction. Variations which do not do so ultimately lead a species to disappear. Groups of similar species which become separated over time, for example by a geographic boundary, may change in different ways, their divergence reflecting their adaptation to their separate and particular local environments. Thus, the challenge of novelty, could be addressed by pointing to these variations, which together constitute a gradual process of change, sifted by natural selection. In the vocabulary of complexity, Darwin's proposals reflect a kind of self-organisation at the level of the organism and at the species level as a result of self-organisation among groups of organisms. Interaction between the organisms and the physical environment could explain the emergence of new behaviour and new forms of organism.[18,19]

But how did these novelties arise? Biologists and philosophers struggled with this problem. Thomas Huxley, writing around the same time as Darwin, disagreed with him. Novelty, Huxley said, emerged in a sudden, discontinuous and unpredicted fashion before natural selection exerted its influence. Huxley postulated that the role of natural selection was to refine the newly and expectedly emergent species.[20] A key contribution which helped clarify the debate came from Mendel's explanation of the genetic basis of inheritance. This allowed people like Bateson to argue that the mutations giving rise to new species typically arose as small changes in genetic material, an idea that was taken up by other scientists, including Fisher, Haldane and Wright in the first half of the twentieth century. From the work of these scientists, the neo-Darwinian perspective emerged, most recently refined by Dawkins.[21] Again, at the risk of oversimplifying, this neo-Darwinian perspective proposes that new forms emerge from the formative influence of competition on variations which occur completely by chance at the level of genes. The competition, which will select which of these transvariations survive, reflects the organism's ability to adapt to its environment. Stacey calls this 'adaptationist teleology', a slightly confusing term which Stacey uses to reflect the notion of a process that forms and influences a species and its organisms in the absence of any predetermined and efficient cause.[22] Once a novel form has emerged, the genetic programme which has predisposed its survival secures its lifetime development, in order to control the development again in future generations in the interests of gene survival through adaptation. Change, Stacey argues, is movement to a stable state of adaptation to the environment.

The influence of mathematics on complexity

Throughout the course of this book many references will be made to the mathematical conventions which have shaped many of the insights in the complexity sciences, particularly in computing. In this section I briefly review the history of mathematics in order to secure a further anchor on the history of thought, and to support the view in this book that exploring complexity sciences for health-care is not inherently novel, but part of a continuing tradition of reflecting on the nature of knowledge.

Mathematics really begins with Plato, for whom mathematics was geometry. Plato's academy in Athens had, above its entrance, an engraved sign saying, 'Let no-one enter here who is unacquainted with geometry'. Up until the time of Galileo, regarded as the father of modern science because he began to carry out systematic experiments using mathematical language, maths was geometry; mathematicians sought answers only in terms of geometrical figures. Several centuries after Plato, the Persians developed a new system of numerical analysis for which they used the Arabic word 'aljabr', which meant binding together. This process involved reducing the number of unknown quantities in a problem by binding them together in an equation. The term became anglicised as 'algebra', which conventionally took the letters from the beginning of the alphabet to stand for various constant numbers. From such simple algebra, higher algebra involving relationships or functions emerged, conventionally denoted by letters taken from the end of the alphabet. For example, $y = x + 1$ is a statement in which the variable y is recognised to be a function of x.[23]

It was Descartes' contribution to bring these two forms of mathematical calculation together, in what schoolboys in the UK now ruefully recognise as Cartesian coordinates. Thus, Descartes could represent in graphical form the above higher function, $y = x + 1$, as a straight line crossing the y axis at the level of 1. Descartes could also graphically represent more complicated functions like $y = x^2$, which takes the form of a parabola. However, what neither Descartes nor Galileo could do was graphically represent the motion of a body at variable speeds, i.e. accelerating or decelerating. This was Newton's contribution with his development of differential calculus, where the term 'differential' indicates the infinitely small difference, for example in velocity, noted in a particular body over time. Newtonian equations became known as differential equations, and his contribution was to represent the notion of the infinite mathematically for the first time.

As Descartes had struggled with the notion of acceleration, so

Newton struggled with a problem which defeated mathematicians up until the beginning of the twentieth century. This was the problem of representing the motion of three bodies under mutual gravitational attraction. Historians of mathematics point to one basic feature of mathematics around that time which represented the major impediment to solving the problem of the three celestial bodies. All the equations in mathematics that were solvable up until the early twentieth century were linear. As Capra points out, whenever non-linear equations appeared, they tended to be linearised, i.e. reduced to insignificant contributions to the problem – small insignificant changes in temperature, shallow irrelevant alterations in wave function.[23] However, biologists were showing that nature was relentlessly non-linear, and when mathematicians addressed non-linearity, some surprising results emerged. Simple deterministic equations produced unsuspected rich and varied behaviour. Complex and at times chaotic behaviour could give rise to order and beauty. Mathematicians quickly realised that exact prediction became impossible, even though the equations were strictly deterministic. More than any other this key feature of non-linearity shifted mathematical appraisal from quantitative to qualitative. But perhaps the most important feature of non-linearity which mathematicians found was self-reinforcing feedback. Consider the simple mathematical function $x \rightarrow Kx(1-x)$. This is a relationship often found in non-linear systems, the evolution of which produces unexpected results. Consider this function when the value of K is 3. The equation now becomes: $x \rightarrow 3x(1-x)$

Consider also that the value of x lies between 0 and 1. Thus, we can think of the value of x stretching along a single line, whose origin is zero and whose terminus is 1. Taking a few points on this line, where $x = 0$, 0.2, 0.4, 0.6, 0.8 and then 1, the equation is solved as follows:

For $x = n$	Solution
$x = 0$	0
$x = 0.2$	0.48
$x = 0.4$	0.72
$x = 0.6$	0.72
$x = 0.8$	0.48
$x = 1$	0

The results show something quite unpredictable and strange. The equation is solved with numbers increasing up to 0.72, and then appears to fold back on itself, back to zero. This is called the Baker transformation and was one of the earliest examples of non-linearity applied to deterministic equations.

However, it was the French mathematician Jules Henri Poincare who made the greatest contribution to the mathematics of complexity in the early part of the twentieth century. His contribution was to revisualise mathematics, inventing a form of visible mathematics called topology which describes the mathematics of relationships. Poincare developed this component of mathematics to analyse qualitative features of complex dynamical problems. In this approach Poincare was the first to solve the celebrated three body problem and in doing so probably described the first chaotic attractor, although he didn't call it such. In the words of Ian Stewart 'Poincare was gazing at the footprints of chaos'.[24]

Pattern and form in the arts

We have illustrated the way in which the history of thought addressed the two notions which are central to this book – the struggle between structure and pattern, the tension being between determinism and unpredictability. However, this debate was not confined to the natural sciences, nor to mathematics. We refer here to two simple illustrations from painting and music which show how artists also struggled with these notions. Both examples are taken from the twentieth century.

The picture illustrated in Plate 1 was painted by Robert Delaunay in 1917 and now sits in the Tate in London. It depicts the view of the Eiffel Tower from the top of the Arc de Triomphe, although it was not painted in the natural setting. We see that Delaunay was beginning to be influenced by the structural properties of the paintings of the more severe cubists like Braque and Picasso, whose exploration of form gave rise to the multi-angle views of structures depicted in the two dimensions of the canvas. Until then Delaunay's painting had been more influenced by the impressionism of Monet and the pointillisme of Seurat. Delaunay had been enchanted by the lyrical use of colour in these schools but felt that the paintings, particularly of the pointillists, lacked solidity and structure. The suggestion of firm geometrical shapes in the painting shows how the artist was struggling with these two notions of pattern arising from colour, and structure delivered by geometrical form.

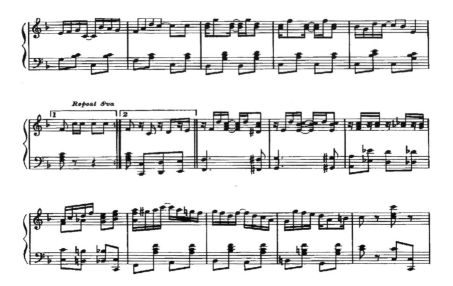

Figure 2.1 Extract from Scott Joplin, *Elite Syncopations*. Reproduced with permission from Joplin (1974).

Figure 2.1 is a small phrase of music taken from Scott Joplin's *Elite Syncopations*, written around the turn of the twentieth century. Joplin's syncopation was a novel musical technique in which the melodic note occurred in the offbeat of the bar. It is relatively easy to see, in this small phrase of music. The structure of the music is delivered by the left hand's constant steady rhythmic beat. The pattern of the semiquavers of the right hand, and their introduction in the offbeat of the note illustrates how Joplin was addressing the juxtaposition of structure (left hand) with pattern (delivered by the right hand).

Conclusion

As healthcare professionals we struggle in our daily work to predict the unpredictable, to explain the inexplicable. Why was this patient

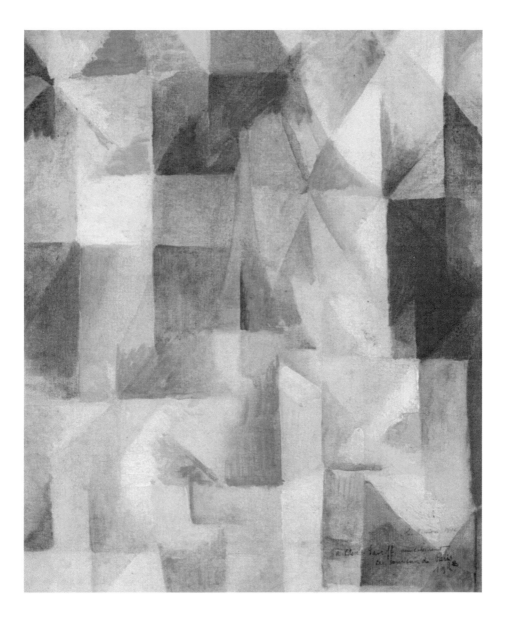

Plate 1 Robert Delaunay (1912) *Window on the City.*
(Reproduced with permission from Lynton N (1980) *The Story of Modern Art.*
Phaidon, Oxford.)

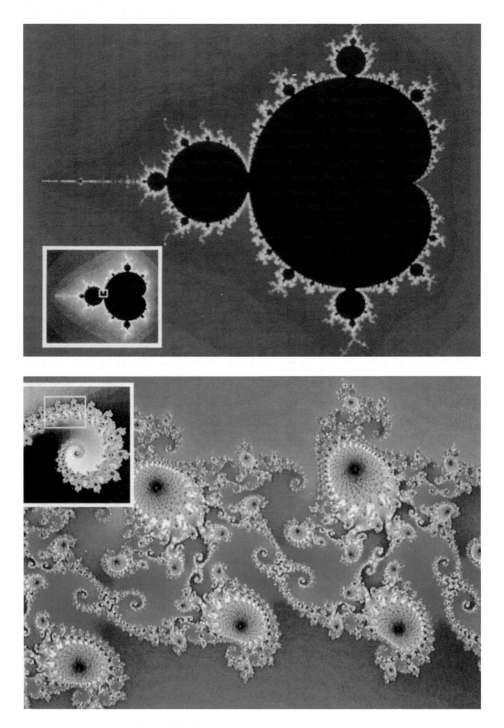

Plate 2 The Mandelbrot Set.
See http://aleph0.clarku.edu/~djoyce/julia/explorer.html for more examples.

the 1 in 200 who developed the serious side-effect of this drug? Why did this particular person, who had an evidence-based diagnosis and was receiving evidence-based treatment, go on to die of her evidence-based disease? Why do some conditions seem so eminently predictable, like the course of a true appendicitis, while others, like the rate of progression of heart failure, appear so elusive to firm predictive strategies? We recognise, with a dreary familiarity, so many occasions when the appropriate infusion of inputs is simply not accompanied by the anticipated outputs. 'If things were that simple', the philosopher Derrida said, 'word would have gotten round'.

In this chapter, I have attempted to point out that healthcare professionals are neither the first, nor the only, group to have experienced these dilemmas. I hope that this brief canter through the history of knowledge in Western civilisation has been enough to at least suggest that mankind has grappled with these kinds of issues since knowledge was recorded. Epicurus and Heraclitus did, as did Aristotle and Plato; our own work in medicine is still influenced by Descartes, Darwin and Kant who joined in and hugely developed the debate. Contemporary artists, poets and musicians still struggle with similar issues in their own disciplines. This is quite simply because the issues are central to the nature of human enquiry. In medicine today we see the frank concession that the linear reductionist model, upon which the majority of our most cherished assumptions lie, is simply not up to the task of addressing either a resolutely non-linear world, or its maddeningly unpredictable inhabitants. More than this, the model can at times be inaccurate and positively misleading.

In the introduction to this chapter I mentioned faddism, and the need to address the accusation that the exploration of complexity is at best light relief from, and at worst a distraction from the expectation that doctors are there to make diagnoses, apply the principles of biomedicine, and generally get on with the battle against disease (an uplifting military metaphor which suggests that doctors and nurses see themselves as courageous foot soldiers engaged in a worthy activity). In response to this I have tried to place our enquiry into complexity firmly in the history of knowledge. Far from participating in novelty for vicarious pleasure, I suggest that medicine is at the cusp of change, confused by the hegemony of science, yet still relying on it; challenged by the non-linearity of an unpredictable world; frustrated at our failed attempts to control the uncontrollable. Complexity offers us an expanded explanatory model, which allows us to retain what is best from the contemporary paradigm, while extending our interpretive potential using its insights.

References

1   Senge P *et al.* (1994) *The Fifth Discipline Handbook.* Nicholas Brealey, London.

2   Bateson G (1979) *Mind and Nature: a necessary unity.* Dutton, New York.

3   Bailey C (1947) *Titus Lucretius Carus de Natura Rerum.* Oxford University Press, Oxford.

4   Popper KR (1963) *The Open Society and Its Enemies.* Princeton University Press, New Jersey.

5   Plato (Translation 1979) *The Sophist.* Garland, New York.

6   Descartes R. See *Meditations Metaphysiques* (1976). J Vrin, Paris.

7   Dixon M and Sweeney K (2000) *The Human Effect in Medicine.* Radcliffe Medical Press, Oxford.

8   Porter R (1997) *The Greatest Benefit to Mankind.* Fontana Press, London.

9   Descartes R (1912) *A Discourse on Method: medication and principles.* Veitch J (translation) Dent & Sons Ltd, London.

10 Greaves D (1996) *Mystery in Western Medicine.* Ashgate Publishing Ltd, Aldershot.

11 Foucault M (1963) *The Birth of the Clinic.* Tavistock, London.

12 Wordsworth W (1947) The Tables Turned. In: *The Poems of Wordsworth.* MacMillan, London.

13 Capra F (1982) *The Turning Point.* Simon and Schuster, New York.

14 Stacey R (2000) *Complexity and Management: fad or radical challenge to systems thinking?* Routledge, London.

15 Windelband W (1901) *A History of Philosophy.* MacMillan, New York.

16 Webster G and Goodwin BC (1982) The origin of species: a structuralist approach. *Journal of Social and Biological Structures.* 5: 15–47.

17 Kant I (1780) *Critique of Judgement. See* Pluhar WS (1987). Hackett, Indianapolis.

18   Darwin C (1859) *The Origin of Species by Means of Natural Selection* or *The Preservation of Favoured Races in the Struggle for Life*. John Murray, London.

19   Darwin C (1871) *The Descent of Man*. John Murray, London.

20   Huxley T (1863) *Man's Place in Nature*. Appleton, New York.

21   Dawkins R (1976) *The Selfish Gene*. Oxford University Press, New York.

22   Stacey R (2000) *Complex Responsive Processes in Organisations*. Routledge, London.

23   Capra F (1996) *The Web of Life: a new scientific understanding of systems*. Anchor Books, New York.

24   Stewart I (1989) *Does God Play Dice?* Blackwell, Cambridge, MA.

25   Joplin S (1974) Reproduced from *Scott Joplin Piano Rags*.

CHAPTER THREE

Clinical knowledge, chaos and complexity

Tim Holt

Summary

This chapter develops the notions of multidimensional phase space, non-linearity, emergence and chaos in the context of clinical medicine. I illustrate the conventional tendency towards 'linearising', that is approximating the complex and unpredictable variations in complex systems to make them seem more linear – and therefore easier to comprehend. Genetic research, often regarded as the epitome of the reductionist approach, is reconsidered from the perspective of complex adaptive systems. The relevance of these ideas to clinical specialties is then discussed, using examples from neurology, cardiology, diabetes and infectious diseases. Heart rate variability, a prerequisite for good health has a fractal structure; variations in blood glucose levels in diabetes can be considered as the trajectory of a chaotic system; and current research into brain physiology supports the view of the mind as an emergent phenomenon. The chapter ends with some comments on complexity and alternative medicine.

Introduction

Clinical knowledge and its use during the consultation has changed dramatically over the past 20 years, both through the extension of research-based evidence into clinical practice, and through the development of novel means of delivery and communication. The introduction of computers into the consulting room provides an almost unlimited supply of information, guidance and opinion. To some this has become an essential facet of the consultation, while for others it remains an unwelcome distraction from the patient–practitioner interface.

In *Civilisation*,[1] an influential work of the late 1960s, Kenneth Clark appealed to us to 'defy all of those forces that threaten to impair our humanity: lies, tanks, tear-gas, ideologies, opinion polls, mechanisation, planners, computers – the whole lot'. However, Clark conceded that *Civilisation*, largely concerning the history of pictorial art, had been conveyed to advantage through a relatively new genre – that of the television serial documentary. The need to retain our integrity and dignity in the face of advancing technology is a challenge for every generation. The movement away from linear and reductionist models in science is a response to this wider sentiment as well as a frank concession, increasingly evident, that such models are inaccurate and often misleading.

In this chapter, some of the models and frameworks on which our clinical knowledge and evidence is based will be explored, and the theories of complexity and chaos examined for insights into ways forward for medicine in the twenty-first century.

Traditional models

Linear thinking is a sort of 'mischief' which creeps into much of the way we conceptualise the world and it displays itself in numerous ways: in the design of randomised control trials, which separate the effect under study from its context and may assume that components vary independently; in the way that outcomes are presumed to be predictable and proportional to the magnitude of the intervention; in the randomisation of study and control groups based on only a small number of matched parameters; in innumerable metabolic unit studies which control essential variables (e.g. exercise, using bedrest); and in the assumption that results (whether positive or negative) can be generalised to a much wider population, with disregard for the cultural and genetic heterogeneity across society.

Statistically speaking, linearity creeps in through the assumption that populations exist on a bell curve with a normal distribution, and through the failure to recognise the interactive nature of causative factors. In the case of variables which cannot be controlled, average values are taken. In addition, there is a tendency to deal with snap-shots of systems which are in fact highly dynamic and change through time, simply because the statistical evaluation of longitudinal time-series data is far more difficult than that based on single cross-sections.

New models and concepts

New strategies for understanding complex systems would need to recognise a number of characteristics often ignored in traditional models. These include:

- multiple dimensions
- non-linearity
- dynamism
- emergence.

Multiple dimensions

Two obstacles to conceptualising complex systems are the three-dimensional world of our everyday experience, and the two-dimensional paper or screen on which relationships are often portrayed. The first cartographers who had to represent the surface of the earth on a flat piece of paper would appreciate this dilemma. Such approximations may work well for short-range needs, but become increasingly distorted when applied globally to the system's whole.

The concept of a *multidimensional space of possibilities* has become increasingly familiar with the introduction of computer search engines and the Internet. If each variable in a system is plotted along an axis within such a space, a vast array of configurations can be represented. Within the space of possible values for the variables of a system, some will be more frequently occupied than others, whilst some may not be accessible. This framework, in which the *actual* is a subset of the *possible*, is an important one in the development of complex modelling strategies. Changes to the specification of a subset may have highly non-linear effects on the outcome.

Box 3.1 Multiple dimensions

The *library of Babel*[2] is an imaginary library which contains *all possible books!* Each contains a finite number of characters on each page. The characters comprise all the letters of the alphabet, as well as commas, full stops, exclamation marks and all the other grammatical symbols. Each book sits 'next to' (in a large but finite number of dimensions) all the other books which differ by only a single character. The library is vast, but finite. Most of the books are non-sense; a small subset are grammatically correct but meaningless. A tiny subset contains meaningful prose, within which can be found all the books which have ever been, and ever will be written, together with even more that will not.

The *library of Mendel*, coined by Daniel Dennett, is a similar array but of genotypes rather than books, specified by the nucleotide bases which comprise nucleic acids. Only a tiny fraction of these genotypes could encode a viable organism, and within this subset is found all the life forms that have ever lived on earth. Some regions may be viable but are not accessible through viable routes. Genetic evolution proceeds in small non-linear steps through this multidimensional space, many steps proving fatal, most of the rest leading ultimately down blind alleys to extinction.

Such models are now more than curious thought experiments. The advent of electronic medical literature indexes and Internet search engines has made the exploration of multidimensional space an everyday activity, and part of the new framework on which our clinical knowledge is based.

The management of raised serum cholesterol is an example in which the recognition of multiple dimensions is helping to overcome conceptual barriers. Protocols for the selection of primary prevention candidates have become more complex over the years, and with this complexity has come better, more rational and more cost-effective care.

The Sheffield table,* which provides guidance on the selection of patients for the measurement and treatment of raised cholesterol, attempts to fit six dimensions (cholesterol level, age, smoking status, presence of diabetes, hypertension, left ventricular hypertrophy) on a flat piece of paper. It avoids the seventh dimension (sex) by giving a separate chart for men and women. The Joint British Societies' table** takes both total and HDL cholesterol levels into account. These diagrams stretch us to our limit of tolerance in pictorialising heart disease risk. Such limited tolerance is inevitable because our paper is two-dimensional. Many of us now rely on computerised risk assessment tools, which would be essential if further variables were to be added. Computers, far from being a threat to our humanity, may enable us to tailor care appropriately simply because of this lack of dimension-limitation. The use of such tools will inevitably become standard practice as the results of the human genome project deliver increasingly complex and individualised knowledge with which to plan the prevention and treatment of disease.

Non-linearity

A *linear* relationship between two variables produces the familiar straight line plot on a Cartesian graph.

The relationship may be described as: $y = ax + c$, where a is the gradient of the line and c is the point of intersection of the line with the y axis (i.e. the value of y when $x = 0$). As x increases, y increases in a predictable way and in direct proportion, because the line is straight (i.e. the gradient a is constant).

A *non-linear* relationship might take the form $y = ax^n + c$ (where n is the power to which the variable x is raised). In general terms, if n does not equal 1, or a is in fact a variable not a constant, the

*The Sheffield table (1995) *Lancet.* **346**: 1467–71.
The Joint British Societies' table (1998) *Heart.* **80: S1–S29.

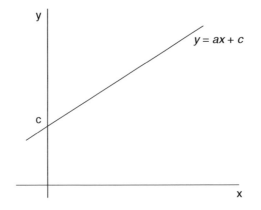

Figure 3.1 Linear relationship.

equation becomes non-linear. As non-linear processes are so common in natural systems, the correct perspective would see the above linear equation $y = ax + c$ as a special case where a is a constant and $n = 1$.

So the inclusion of powered terms, or the presence of two variables multiplied together creates non-linearity in a relationship, a subject discussed further in Chapter 4. The behaviour of a system and our ability to predict outcomes becomes fundamentally changed when non-linear processes are involved (Box 3.2).

Box 3.2 Non-linearity

Imagine the difficulty faced by an investor predicting the interest returns over the coming year on a bank account offering compound interest (a non-linear relationship between sums invested and interest accrued) compared with a simple interest account (in which the interest is directly proportional to the time spent in the account). Imagine how much difference the timing of deposits and withdrawals makes to the prediction of returns on the compound interest account, where error in measurement of any of the invested or withdrawn sums becomes amplified by the non-linearity. Now imagine that the interest rate varies, so that as well as having a raised power term, there are two variables multiplied together. Finally, imagine introducing further non-linearities: the interest rate offered is related to the balance of the account, so that higher savings attract a greater interest rate, and in the long term is partly dependent on the total amount of invested capital the bank holds.

There is nothing fanciful in this discussion – it is the way real bank accounts often work, and yet we are tempted to cut the otherwise daunting process of prediction down to size using the following approximations:

- assume that the compound interest is in fact simple interest
- take an average for the variable interest rate during the period (i.e. make it a constant)
- assume that the relationship between interest rate and balance is itself linear
- assume that the processes influencing the variables are unconnected with each other.

In making these assumptions, we are following a long and often subconscious tradition through which complex systems are made 'understandable' though linear approximation. The above example is a very simple one based on a few variables. Imagine how much more difficult it is to predict the behaviour of complex physiological and sociological systems, and how inadequate the linear approximations then become.

Dynamism

A dynamical system can be represented in a *phase space* of possible values for the variables. Because the system may tend to settle in certain regions of this space, it contains *attractors*. The form and structure of these attractors, discussed in Chapter 2, are essential features of the system's dynamics.

The assumption is frequently made that the statistical properties of a system will remain basically the same over extended time periods, when in reality such properties may be *non-stationary*. The difficulties in interpreting time-series data are discussed by Glass and Kaplan,[3] and involve new terms such as *bifurcation*, the phenomenon whereby a system's attractor changes form or behaviour quite abruptly. Bifurcation has become an essential term in non-linear dynamics, and will be discussed below in the cardiology and diabetes sections.

A step forward in understanding and interpreting time-series data has come through the use of neural networks, adaptive software units which consist of input and output layers between which a *hidden layer* (or layers) modifies the transmission of incoming information. The hidden layer processes this information by attributing 'weights' to different input patterns, and the weights are adjusted according to the ongoing experience of the system through feedback of emerging results. Such a feedback process is complex and very difficult to understand using reductionist approaches. However, neural network software can adapt to the non-stationary properties of the system. Neural networks have become a basic building block of artificial intelligence systems, and are likely to feature prominently in medical practice in the future.

Emergence

An essential feature of complex systems which linear models ignore is *emergence*, the phenomenon by which new properties arise through the complex interactions and connectivity of lower-level processes.

Beneath the surface of complex systems there are often remarkably simple processes at work. John Holland has explored the simple rule-based models involved in the design of board games, and found that emergent effects arise remarkably easily. Human players have hardly touched the vast space of all possible chess games. The algorithms that produce the emergent strategies of chess-playing computers cannot do so by exploring the extent of this space during a game. Instead, they rely on programmed rules, exploration of regions of the space close to the current position, and learning in response to the strategies of the human opponent and the relative successes of their own moves. Such a model provides a dramatic example of emergent behaviour within a bounded and constrained rule-based system of sequential interactions.

Echo is a programme designed by Holland to represent the features common to a wide spectrum of complex adaptive systems, including the local interaction of component agents and learning from past experiences. The design of Echo is described in Holland's book, *Hidden Order: how adaptation builds complexity*,[4] and borrows the principles of information storage, mutation, interaction and replication from genetics.

Genetics represents a frequently quoted example of the success of reductionism, since the discovery in 1959 of the double helix structure of DNA, leading much more recently to the completion of the human genome project. But a realistic picture of the complexity of gene functioning recognises the interdependence of multiple gene activities (Box 3.3).

Box 3.3 The genetic model

- Genes cannot function outside the biochemical context in which they are embedded.
- Single genes may be attributable to specific functions, but they are dependent on other genes and cellular enzymes to regulate their own functioning.
- These enzymes are again dependent for their production and activation on genes, including in many cases the genes they are regulating.
- A complex web of interactions between genes, their activators, suppressors, substrates and products maintains the system far from equilibrium as an interdependent network of self-regulating feedback cycles.
- There is tension and paradox present: a single gene may produce both deleterious and beneficial effects to the organism.
- Changes in a gene's structure or functioning changes the context for the other genes.
- A very small genetic change can have disproportionate effects on the organism's phenotype.

Such a model, already familiar to medical practitioners, may be more widely applicable in the field of healthcare.

An example might be drug interactions, which are almost always attributed to a combination of two drugs, A and B. Rarely are we advised that A interacts with B only if drug C is also prescribed, and yet there is good reason to suppose that much more complex interactions are commonplace. The National Service Framework for Older People recognises the need to closely monitor patients on multiple therapies. When taking more than four drugs the 'space of possible drug combinations' is vast and a specific combination (representing a point in this space) may have only been 'visited' by a small number of individuals, none of whom have been included in a trial of drug interactions.

The increasingly common scenario in which the patient arrives to see the practitioner with printouts from the Internet, giving detail which leaves the practitioner's knowledge far behind, emphasises the need for *context* in learning and education. Genes cannot function without context, and knowledge is worth little without it either. Working with the patient and combining the respective educational frameworks produces a new, richer context in which the information supplied by the patient becomes useful to both parties. Similarly, isolated items of information provided through decision-support software (and usually contributed by specialists in piecemeal fashion) may leave parts of our own knowledge isolated from appropriate context. The cross-referencing capabilities of computerised resources (including hyperlinking) are a valuable means of offsetting this risk, creating fluidity not just physically between educational material sources, but also cognitively between the various compartments of an individual's knowledge base.

The volume of information available to both practitioners and patients is now so vast that no individual can hope to encompass more than an outline of it. The emphasis on medical education is shifting in response to this realisation towards a facilitating role for generalist clinicians, who must come to terms with the ultimate limitations of their knowledge base and use their training and experience to access the appropriate information from reliable, up-to-date sources.

Clinical applications of chaos theory

The application of non-linear dynamics requires a number of new terms, described in the previous chapter, which can be used to analyse the time-series data of physiological variables. Some of the statistical techniques involved are quite different from traditional linear methods. These are described briefly in Box 3.4, but a deeper understanding may be gained from reading some of the references listed below.[3,5]

Box 3.4 Non-linear time-series analysis

Non-linear time-series analysis frequently involves the recon-struction of an attractor, through the plotting of data in a phase space diagram. Such a diagram may involve numerous variables (x, y, z, etc.) each represented by its own coordinate axis, with the state of the system at any given time represented by a point in this space. In a weather system, x, y and z might be the air temperature, pressure and humidity at a certain location. In a medical scenario, the coordinates might be blood glucose, insulin and glucagon levels in an individual.

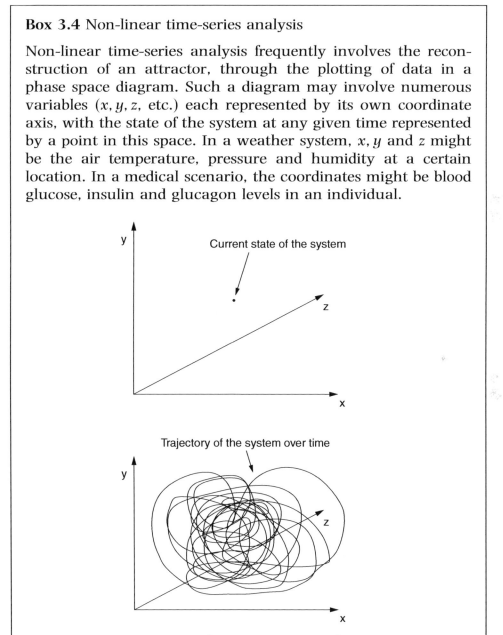

Fig 3.2 Non-linear time-series analysis.

Alternatively, the diagram may involve just one variable x, with each subsequent coordinate axis representing the value of the variable after successive time delays: $x_{(t)}$, $x_{(t+1)}$, $x_{(t+2)}$, $x_{(t+3)}$, etc. This technique is called *data embedding*.

In the simplest form, the graph would be a two-dimensional plot of $x_{(t)}$ against $x_{(t+1)}$ for each value of $x_{(t)}$. Whilst random variation produces no pattern, *chaos* may produce a single-humped one-dimensional curve.

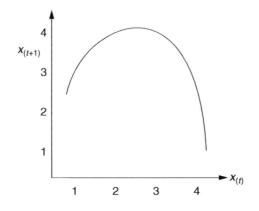

Figure 3.3 Data embedding.

Attractors may take various forms. *Point* attractors, *periodic* attractors, and the *strange attractors* of chaotic systems display different patterns in phase space. A slice through an attractor produces a *Poincare section* or return mapping, which is a plane recurrently bisected by the system's trajectory.

The trajectories within a chaotic system tend to diverge from close starting points, displaying *sensitivity to initial conditions*. This tendency is measurable as a *Lyapunov exponent*, which is positive in a chaotic system.

Random noise has no attractor, takes up all of phase space, is infinite in its dimensions and does not have a positive Lyapunov exponent.

Chaos has a finite dimension number and reveals the under-lying order by confining the system to a *strange attractor*: it has the fractal properties of self-similarity and a dimension number which is typically *non-integer* (e.g. 2.3, 3.4). The attractor's dimension may be different from the number of variables which influence it and it can be calculated using the embedded time-series data of a single variable.

The distinction between chaos and random noise may seem academic, but it is crucial to the understanding of the system's basic dynamics, and reveals the true source of variation. The underlying *determinism* of chaotic variation allows a degree of short-range prediction to be made, provided the dimension number is low.[5] In medicine, this distinction has implications for the measurement of physiological parameters, for the understanding of disease patterns and for the control of disordered physiological mechanisms.

In order to extend these principles into medical practice, we will take examples from five areas: cardiology, diabetes, neurology, infectious disease and critical care.

Cardiology

Cardiology provides a good example of where the principles of chaos theory have led to a revision of basic assumptions about the underlying models.

Heart rate variability has been shown to have fractal structure and to be required for healthy cardiovascular function. A reduction in variability conveys a poorer prognosis following acute myocardial infarction and may be associated with aborted Sudden Infant Death Syndrome (SIDS). Whilst these associations are not necessarily causal (and in the case of myocardial infarction probably reflect altered autonomic tone as a cause for both), they demonstrate that variability is often a feature of healthy systems rather than diseased ones.

Goldberger and colleagues have discussed the fractal structure of the His-Purkinje conduction network, and investigated the role of the atrioventricular node not in passively conducting impulses arising from the sinus node and providing a back-up pacemaker, but in actively generating activity which combines with that of the sinus node to produce a more complex underlying pattern of atrial excitation and ventricular activation.[6] The authors also discuss the possible periodic dynamics underlying ventricular fibrillation.

There is still controversy over the relevance of *chaos* in cardiac arrhythmias, but the phenomenon of *bifurcation*, in which the behaviour of the attractor changes form or structure abruptly, is now a well-studied phenomenon in experimental cardiology. Such bifurcation may involve doubling of the period of a periodic attractor, or the change from periodic to chaotic behaviour. The sequence of period doublings, which has been well studied in ecological systems, has also been demonstrated in myocardial tissue.

An elaborate application of chaos theory to cardiology has been the development of a 'chaotic control' strategy for restoring arrhythmias back to periodic beating in *in vitro* myocardium. This involves the plotting of the beat-to-beat interval against the subsequent interval as a phase space diagram.[7] Within this diagram it is then possible to identify *stable manifolds*, directions in phase space which naturally take the system back towards the desired periodic point (at which the intervals are all the same). Electrical impulses (similar to pacing spikes) then nudge the system back towards the stable manifolds rather than aiming it directly towards the desired point, as this leads to overshooting.

Such a strategy requires three essential elements which might be more widely useful in other areas of medicine:

- frequent monitoring with appropriate feedback
- identification of stable manifolds in phase space
- ongoing feedback of results in order to detect movement of the stable manifolds over time.

Candidates for such a strategy would therefore require a combination of sensors and effectors, appropriate coupling between the two and the ability to learn through feedback of recent results. This is reminiscent of the neural network model described above.

Diabetes

It is not difficult to draw on the principles of complexity theory to model the day-to-day life of a person with diabetes, particularly a type 1 patient on insulin. Such people are only too familiar with the concepts of uncertainty, unpredictability and even *chaos*. The central variable, blood glucose, is determined by numerous factors (insulin doses, carbohydrate intake, exercise level, etc.) which interact through non-linear processes, and the entire system could be represented by a multidimensional phase space of possible values for these variables. The state of the system at any given time could be plotted as a point within this space, and the *trajectory* of this point through time would describe an *attractor* for that person. The attractor might be orderly at times (showing little variability or *periodicity*, if the system tended to return to the same place regularly), but at other times might show chaotic tendencies (for instance during a febrile illness). Treated type 1 diabetes is not simply a condition of insulin deficiency; it is a condition of mismatch between insulin availability and immediate insulin requirement, due to a loss of the negative feedback loop which regulates blood glucose in the normal physiological state. Insulin-injecting behaviour and associated decision making become essential components of the attractor and cannot be separated from the physiology. To complicate matters further, the behavioural response of an individual whose blood glucose is rising may cause lethargy and exercise avoidance, making the level rise higher, creating a situation of positive feedback. The combination of *positive* and *negative feedback* within the attractor of a person with diabetes sets the scene for the *stretch and fold* geometry typical of chaotic systems.

Such a non-linear model has been proposed in an attempt to introduce the principles of chaos theory into diabetes care.[8] In support of this idea, it is interesting to note the following:

- chaos, in its mathematical sense of unpredictable behaviour arising in a low-dimensional system of deterministic but non-linear processes, has been demonstrated even within non-diabetic profiles
- the statistical properties of a patient's profile may be *non-stationary*, i.e. they may show tendencies to vary over time
- as with weather systems, there is a limit to the predictive *horizon* over which the behaviour of the profile can be forecast
- models designed to interpret blood glucose profiles have needed to recognise the non-linear, as well as the non-stationary, properties of the attractor

- such models can often make successful interpretations based on relatively simple underlying rules, a hallmark of complex systems.

How might these principles be used in a practical way to improve the care of people with diabetes?

1 The emphasis in decision making might move away from the practitioner and towards the patient. An individual patient's familiarity with their attractor's properties is likely to be a more enduring guide for blood glucose control than the specific advice offered by practitioners in clinics based on historical blood glucose profiles, as such advice may not remain valid for very long. Motivating patients to learn these properties and adapt to changes in them becomes crucial.

2 Patients may benefit from close monitoring, but only if they are able to respond to emerging results appropriately, thereby restoring the feedback control loop which is broken in type 1 diabetes.

3 Patients may benefit from monitoring even though insulin doses are rarely altered. Impulsive adjustments may exacerbate chaotic tendencies.

4 Decision making and associated behaviour is multidimensional and must take account of the systems *direction* as well as its current state. In the same way as described above in the cardiology section, a tightly controlled patient may intuitively identify *stable manifolds* in phase space and nudge the system towards these manifolds rather than towards the desired point itself. Aiming the system towards the desired point by the quickest possible route will lead to worse control, not better. This same principle has been used to design improved sliding scale protocols for use on labour wards.

5 Changes in the attractor's behaviour might occur quite abruptly as a *bifurcation*. Such a change is a system-wide phenomenon, although it may result from an alteration to a single control parameter. Such a concept may lead to an improved understanding of the variation in control observed at certain times, such as during intercurrent illness, or when other medication such as steroids are prescribed.

6 Above all, the non-linear model recognises that 'wild cards' will

be dealt from time to time, and perhaps allow the patient to accept and live with the uncertainty and unpredictability which exists even in a system which is broadly understandable.

Neurology

Brain physiology is highly non-linear. Such non-linearity is a prerequisite for its emergent properties, including learning, memory, cognition and consciousness. A neurological system based on linear relationships (if it could exist at all) would be capable of little more than reflex actions in response to external stimuli. In reality such reflexes are themselves often highly non-linear. Holland has demonstrated the emergence of three basic properties (reverberation, indefinite memory, anticipation) using a very basic model of neuronal connections which makes only a small number of assumptions about neurone behaviour.[9]

Reverberation is the establishment of cyclical patterns of pulses within such a network, and represents a periodic attractor for the system. Such an attractor pattern is a highly ordered emergent property, but may leave the system unable to respond when requirements change, and the property of neuronal *fatigue* protects the system from this fate.

There has been much debate about whether the brain's attractor exists in the chaotic realm. Certainly the system as a whole relies on non-linearity to adapt to new demands and learn from past experiences. Memory and learning are highly adaptive. As a compromise, cortical functioning must be kept a safe distance from the orderly realm and this leaves it prone to instabilities which may underlie numerous physical and psychiatric disease states. Scott Barton has discussed the implications for psychological mechanisms resulting from this need to achieve both stability and flexibility and the possible insights that chaos theory might offer.[10]

The effect of ethanol on brain physiology has been modelled in terms of a reduction in non-linearity towards linearity.[11] Once again non-linearity is a feature of healthy, adaptive physiology. Disease processes are all too often framed in terms of disordered receptor activity or chemical imbalance and rarely in terms of disordered dynamics, perhaps because such models lend themselves more readily to simple solutions provided by the pharmaceutical industry. The elucidation of dynamical patterns and mechanisms might in fact open doors to new therapeutic approaches in neurology, psychiatry and elsewhere.

The electroencephalogram (EEG) is a well-studied representation of brain dynamics and an obvious target for the application of the principles of chaos theory.[12] Studies of EEGs have attempted to identify chaos through the reconstruction of the underlying attractor, which can then be examined and its chaotic properties detected if present. Such properties would include a positive *Lyapunov exponent* (a measure of the tendency for trajectories to diverge from close starting points in phase space) and *fractal* geometry which includes a non-integer dimension number and self-similar structure at different magnifications. Disease states may be represented by excursions towards the orderly realm, as seen in the periodic patterns typical of EEGs in both petit-mal epilepsy and Creutzfeldt-Jakob disease.

Whilst these observations are of diagnostic rather than therapeutic importance, it has also been suggested that the principles of chaos theory might enable seizure activity to be anticipated before the seizure actually happens, through a deeper understanding of the underlying dynamics.[13] It is the abruptness of onset of abnormal seizure activity which restricts the lives of so many people with epilepsy, and leaves them dependent on often toxic medication. Whilst unpredictability is a hallmark of chaotic systems, broad patterns may be identifiable (as they clearly are in weather systems) which may allow predictions to be made, suggesting a way forward for the development of novel therapeutic techniques.

Infectious disease

William Schaffer has described the consequences of the introduction of non-linear dynamics into both ecology and disease epidemiology:[14]

'...the equilibrium view of the world central to two decades of theorising would go forever out of the window. In particular, it would no longer make sense to think of such systems in terms of a balance between intrinsic forces, forever searching out some mythical attracting point, and environmental vagaries perturbing the system away from it.'

This shift in perspective could potentially alter both our statistical evaluation of disease patterns and our approach to disease control. In the case of measles, it has been possible to examine the North American data from before the days of vaccination, when the illness was a common infection that few children escaped. Schaffer describes the *'seasonally forced SEIR'* model, which can be summarised as follows. The population is divided into four groups in terms of stages of measles infection:

S – *Susceptible* Children are born into this group (ignoring transient maternal antibody protection)
E – *Exposed* (but not yet infective)
I – *Infective*
R – *Recovered* (and immune for the rest of life).

Individuals enter group S by being born, leave any group by dying and, in most cases, move through these groups in succession. Movement between the groups can be described using three differential equations. The movements are mutually dependent, because a high level of infected individuals will accelerate the movement between groups S and E, creating a positive feedback amplification loop. Other variables involved include the total population size, the natural birth and death rates and the frequency of contact between individuals in the community, which varies partly according to seasonal temperature.

This model has its limitations (and in itself involves some linear assumptions, such as constant population sizes and uniform life expectancy), but it creates a low-dimension system of interdependent variables whose behaviour is non-linear. The dynamics can be plotted in a phase space diagram and an attractor can be constructed. This can then be used to test competing hypotheses over the appropriate underlying model. In the case of measles, Schaffer argues that a combination of cycles and chaos sustained by seasonal variation in contact rates fits the data better than an endemic equilibrium state disrupted by noise. Much of the variation is therefore an emergent property of the system and not a result of external influences (e.g. inward migration of measles virus from outside the community). Such an insight (only possible by applying non-linear techniques) gives a truer picture of the under-lying dynamics, and might enable maximum infection rates to be predicted within closer limits, and vaccination programmes to be planned more effectively.

Critical care

Seely and Christou have applied the principles of non-linear dynamics to the intensive care scenario, in which patients frequently die from Multiple Organ Dysfunction Syndrome (MODS). Attempts to target therapies towards single mediators of the host response to trauma and sepsis have been ineffective, because they fail to recognise the *connectivity* between the multiple processes involved, which include immune, metabolic, endocrine and neural responses. The authors discuss the potential use of non-linear models, which would take account of the dynamism in the system, as well as the interdependence of the variables and disease mechanisms involved.[15]

Alternative and complementary medicine

Alternative therapies are often paradoxical in their mechanisms. Needles are inserted to relieve pain, tender joints are manipulated until they click, those with asthma are told to breathe less often and homoeopathic remedies, which involve the same substances that would normally trigger the symptoms, are diluted to make them stronger. It is little wonder that a major obstacle to their acceptance has simply been lack of *plausibility*.

Also, the methods used in alternative practice are difficult to investigate using standard research designs. It is difficult to organise a double-blind placebo group in a trial of osteopathy or acupuncture, and the remedies prescribed by homoeopaths are often tailored to specific individual characteristics which make it difficult to compare treatment and control groups matched for all these parameters.

In 1983 the Research Council for Complementary Medicine (RCCM) was set up to promote research and encourage safe practice in this field. Some of the work of the RCCM is described in the Royal College of Physicians 1998 booklet, *Science based complementary medicine.*[16]

Included in this publication is a chapter exploring the possible mechanisms of action of homoeopathy, which involves repeated dilutions of 'Mother Tinctures' with vigorous shaking ('succession') between each dilution. Homoeopathic remedies are so dilute that there is probably not a single molecule of 'Mother Tincture' left in a vial of the final product. Any beneficial effect beyond placebo must be due to some sort of memory or information storage imparted by the preparation process on the water molecules themselves, either through their vibrational characteristics or orientation. It is suggested that the repeated dilutions might act in a similar way to the iteration of a fractal such as the Mandelbrot set, which reveals finer and finer detail at each iteration (*see* Plate 2). If a similar process were responsible at the molecular level for the reorientation of water molecules, it begins to become plausible that such altered arrangements might then trigger responses at cell membranes or through immune mediators.

Advocates of homoeopathy are still a little way from demonstrating these effects to general satisfaction, for whilst there is evidence that homoeopathy is better than placebo in a good number of trials, no double-blind trial has found higher dilutions to be more efficacious than less diluted preparations of the same remedy. However, if chaos theory could provide insights which made the mechanism *plausible*, this barrier would be removed and the research funding might follow. It would then be up to the researchers to discover whether or not these effects do indeed occur and whether such therapies should be given a more prominent role in clinical medicine.

Conclusion

The application of non-linear dynamics and complexity theory in medicine has questioned the adequacy of traditional linear models and provided alternative means through which disease patterns and physiological mechanisms can be understood. Such a shift in perspective, coinciding with and made possible by advancing computer technology, should lead to more sensitive means of healthcare delivery as well as novel therapies in a wide range of clinical areas, just a few of which have been explored in this chapter. As a basis for a fundamental rethink across the whole spectrum of medicine, from conceptual modelling to research methodology and clinical practice, these theories surely offer the brightest way forward for the harnessing of twenty-first century technology in the pursuit and protection of human health.

References

1   Clark K (1969) *Civilisation*. BBC, London.

2   Dennett D (1995) *Darwin's Dangerous Idea*. Penguin, London.

3   Glass L and Kaplan D (1993) Time series analysis of complex dynamics in physiology and medicine. *Medical Progress through Technology*. **19**: 115–28.

4   Holland JH (1995) *Hidden Order: how adaptation builds complexity*. Perseus Books, Cambridge, MA.

5   Skinner JE (1994) Low dimensional chaos in biological systems. *Bio/Technology*. **12**: 596–600.

6   Goldberger AL and West BJ (1987) Applications of non-linear dynamics to clinical cardiology. *Annals of the New York Academy of Sciences*. **504**: 195–213.

7   Garfinkel A, Spano ML, Ditto WL and Weiss JN (1992) Controlling cardiac chaos. *Science*. **257**: 1230–5.

8   Holt TA (2002) A chaotic model for tight diabetes control. *Diabetic Medicine*. **19(4)**: 274–8.

9   Holland JH (1998) *Emergence: from chaos to order*. Oxford University Press, Oxford.

10   Barton S (1994) Chaos, self-organisation and psychology. *American Psychologist*. **49**: 5–14.

11   Ehlers CL, Havstad J, Prichard D and Theiler J (1998) Low doses of ethanol reduce evidence for non-linear structure in brain activity. *Journal of Neuroscience*. **18**: 7474–86.

12   Pradhan N and Narayana Dutt D (1993) A nonlinear perspective in understanding the neurodynamics of EEG. *Computers in Biology and Medicine*. **23**: 425–42.

13   Elger CE and Lehnertz K (1998) Seizure prediction by non-linear time series analysis of brain electrical activity. *European Journal of Neuroscience.* **10**: 786–9.

14   Schaffer WM (1985) Can non-linear dynamics elucidate mechanisms in ecology and epidemiology? *IMA Journal of Mathematics Applied in Medicine and Biology.* **2**: 221–52.

15   Seely AJE and Christou NV (2000) Multiple organ dysfunction syndrome: exploring the paradigm of complex non-linear systems. *Critical Care Medicine.* **28**: 2193–200.

16   Meade T (ed.) (1998) *Science Based Complementary Medicine.* Royal College of Physicians, London.

CHAPTER FOUR

Complexity and the clinical encounter

Alan Hassey

'If things were simple, word would have gotten round.'

Derrida (1988)[1]

Summary

Models of the clinical encounter have been developed in general practice over the last 50 years. More recently, there has been an emphasis on the use of probabilistic research evidence in clinical practice. The consultation may usefully use such evidence but the majority of consultations tackle health issues where it may be more useful to consider the patient as a complex system interacting with their environment, where outcome can not be reliably predicted. The patient's narrative of their illness brings the time dimension and the patient's context to the consultation. In addition, there can be flashes of understanding that emerge through the interaction of the doctor and patient. Complexity theory provides a framework for incorporating non-linear science, including narrative and intuition, into clinical practice along with probabilistic forms of evidence. Such a framework raises questions about how, and for what benefit, clinical data is recorded in this age of electronic health records.

Introduction

The essential skills of the clinician are the ability to gain rapport with the patient, to elicit significant findings and to integrate them into an appropriate diagnostic and therapeutic model based on the application of expert clinical methods.[2] Thus clinical medicine is not just a scientific discipline, but depends on expert clinical interpretation and integration of the various contextual narratives that make up the patient's story.[3]

The interaction between patient and clinician has been especially well studied in the context of British general practice through analysis of the patient–doctor consultation. In this chapter I will review the major studies and models of the patient–doctor consultation that have been developed since general practice emerged as a specialty in its own right in the 1950s. I will then review the strengths and weaknesses of applying linear models in the consultation and, finally, consider the application of ideas developed from complexity theory to the clinical encounter. The patient and the clinician can both be seen as complex biological systems living within larger complex systems that make up the local community and society at large. Their interaction over time through various clinical and social encounters may be seen as a complex medico-social system in its own right. How might complexity theory shed new light on the consultation in clinical medicine?

Modelling the clinical encounter (consultation)

The study of what happens in the consultation between clinician and patient has developed in the UK from the 1950s onwards. Balint's work in the 1950s based on case study analysis had a profound influence on the teaching of a generation of British general practitioners (GPs).[4] In the 1960s, Berne developed the transactional analysis model of interactions between individuals.[5] While in the 1970s Byrne and Long published their well-researched and pioneering study of doctors' verbal behaviour.[6] These attempts to develop an understanding of the clinical encounter underpinned the emergence of general practice as a medical specialty in its own right and helped to foster an intellectual, academic and educational framework for the learning and teaching of general practice in the UK.[7]

Roger Neighbour states that the purpose of modelling the consultation is to simplify the complex – 'when we speak about models of some complex experience, we are in the realm of metaphor, of analogy, of maps and representations ... Models make sense of sensation'.[8] Neighbour describes many different models of illness, which include scientific, moral, magical, social and political themes. Some or all of these may come into play during the consultation, both from the patient and the clinician as they seek to make sense of the world. Understanding each other's models of illness is a crucial step on the way to establishing rapport in the clinical encounter.

Early attempts at developing an understanding of the consultation used the 'role model' to study the doctor–patient relationship. An example of a behaviour derived from this model is the 'sick role'. Patients and doctors have certain expectations of each other based on the roles they assume during the consultation. This type of approach tended to reinforce a medical model of illness which was doctor-centred and linked to the achievement of particular tasks during the consultation, while Helman's 'folk model' of illness offered a series of patient-centred tasks during the consultation. Byrne and Long analysed the range of behaviours used by doctors talking to patients and used this model to develop profiles of doctors' consulting styles. All contributed to the development of an understanding of the behaviours and approaches that clinicians could adopt to facilitate the patient–doctor relationship and enhance the quality of the consultation. Neighbour draws on all these influences in the development and presentation of his ideas of a 'left brain organiser' and 'right brain responder', representing the intellectual and intuitive skills respectively which the doctor needs in the consultation.

The rationale for the development of these models has been to progress our knowledge and understanding of the tasks and behaviours in the clinical encounter. Thus it should become easier to learn and teach consultation skills based on an understanding of the tasks and behaviours that facilitate successful outcomes from the consultation. The application of these skills is formally assessed in British general practice, both through the summative assessment of all GP registrars at the end of their training and by the

Royal College of General Practitioners in their examination for membership.

Linear models in clinical practice

The application of an evidence-based approach to medicine is at the heart of recent health policy in the UK.[9] The approach suggests that:

- to make better decisions, clinicians will need to develop the necessary skills and tools to apply probabilistic methods to clinical reasoning[10]
- the application of simple linear models can significantly improve diagnostic performance
- the gathering of good base-rate data in clinical practice and the application of Bayesian statistical techniques[11] could facilitate the application of these methods to clinical care.

If most of our work in clinical practice was effectively modelled using simple linear methods then the adoption of an evidence-based probabilistic approach to clinical care and the consultation would surely be an ethical duty and priority for all practising clinicians. However, Tudor Hart has observed that many patients in primary care do not have the sort of hypertension (raised blood pressure) that lends itself to a standard evidence-based guideline.[12]

The application of a (Popperian) scientific hypothetico-deductive clinical method would seem to be appropriate for the practice of probabilistic, evidence-based medicine. However, there is evidence that expert clinicians do not often use these hypothetico-deductive methods of reasoning.[13] Experts may instead rely on a rich network of factual knowledge (syntax) and the abstract interrelationships between these items (semantics) to make decisions. This highly elaborate, structured and complex knowledge base is the true mark of the expert in the field.[14] So, while it is important to apply linear models where they can enhance clinical performance, it is equally important to understand their limitations.

Patients also use simple linear models to help them understand health and illness. Perhaps the best known of these is the cause–effect model. Examples of this include smoking causing cancer, drugs causing side effects and life events causing depression. Patients may understand the limitations of these models, particularly in their ability to be predictive for the individual, and the importance of social and environmental factors.[15] The use of linear models by the medical profession may well reinforce patient attempts to develop a similar 'scientific' approach to health and illness which will tend to be linear and positivist. These models may provide a useful way for patients to understand health matters. In a time of crisis or serious illness, where there is fear and uncertainty, the apparent certainty of medical science can be reassuring. However, overreliance on linear medical models can cause distress when the apparent certainty does not come about.

So it seems that while linear models can improve our clinical performance they do not reflect the way that expert clinicians make decisions, nor do they necessarily fit easily with the illness profiles and expectations that patients present to their doctors.

Key concepts in complexity theory

Key concepts in complexity theory that I will be using in the remainder of the chapter are as follows.

1 A complex system cannot be understood by analysing its components (reductionism). A system that can be understood in this way is merely complicated (e.g. a jumbo jet). Complexity arises from the interaction between the components of a system and the interaction between the system and its environment.[16] These relationships shift and change over time, often as a result of self-organisation. This can result in new features (emergent properties). The brain, language and the economy are all complex systems. Chaotic systems usually appear from the non-linear interaction of small numbers of components, while complex systems contain a large number of interacting components. Simple theories (or definitions) cannot adequately explain complex systems. Perhaps the best working definition of complexity is by Luhman, 'A complex system contains more possibilities than can be actualised'. [16]

2 It is possible to model complex systems, but these models must themselves be as complex as the systems they represent (e.g. neural networks). Complex systems depend not only on their constituent parts, but also on the interactions between those parts. Thus a reductionist approach to analysis will inevitably lose some of this richness. We can model, explore and explain complex systems – but we may not be able to *understand* them.

3 Complexity is not located at a specific site in a system because it arises from the interaction between the components of the system. Complexity shows itself at the level of the system and many of these systems are biological. Self-organisation is a characteristic of complex systems. These systems are not stable, but tend towards *'self-organised criticality'*, whereby the system organises itself to be maximally sensitive to its environment. Small changes can lead to large differences in outcomes (as in chaotic systems). This sensitivity may be manifested through positive feedback loops, amplifying the effects of change, while negative feedback loops tend to lead to homeostasis.

4 A complex system must also have two key capabilities:
   • it must be able to store information about its environment for future use (representation). This representation may be distributed across the system, existing in the pattern of connections between elements of the system
   • it must be able to adapt its structure when necessary (self-organisation). A system can develop a complex structure from fairly unstructured beginnings.

5 The concept of phase space is taken from chaos theory. A phase space diagram represents the complete set of knowledge about a system over time. It is like a road map of all the possibilities for that system with its history charted as a trajectory through time. Attractors live within phase spaces and represent boundary conditions for the system. Small changes within the system may lead to large and unpredictable changes as the system flips between various stable states (bifurcation).

Complexity and the consultation

Where in the application of linear models is there a place for the unstructured problems that patients present to their doctors, which do not fit easily within an evidence-based approach, or for the intuitive insights and Balint-like 'flashes' of understanding[3] that doctors are suddenly aware of in the consultation? How can we develop an understanding of the everyday clinical practice of a primary care physician, and develop a model for the consultation that reflects the real nature of the clinical encounter? One way of modelling the content of primary care is to use a Stacey diagram.[17]

In the Stacey diagram (Figure 4.1), the zone at the bottom left represents medical conditions for which there is a high degree of certainty and agreement about actions and their effects on outcomes. As our evidence base expands, more conditions should

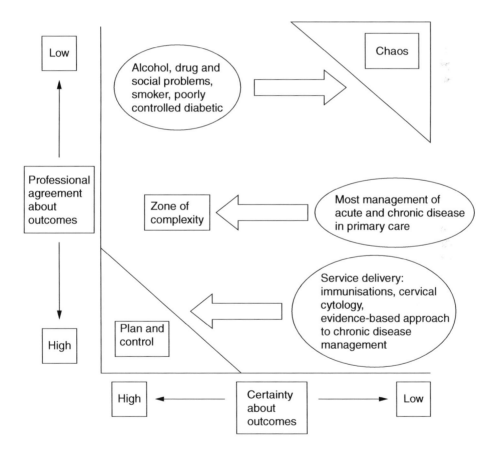

Figure 4.1 The Stacey diagram – the health zone of complexity in primary care. (The word chaos in this diagram is used with the common meaning not the specific meaning in mathematics describing 'chaotic systems'.)

move to the bottom left zone. A linear, evidence-based approach is likely to be appropriate for managing these types of conditions. This zone typically represents a population-based approach to service delivery. The zone in the top right of the diagram represents areas in which agreement and certainty about outcomes is low. There is unlikely to be any (good) evidence to apply to conditions that fall into this zone and a scientific, linear approach is unlikely to be successful. The middle zone represents 'the zone of complexity' where there are only modest levels of agreement and certainty. This applies to individual patients and populations within primary care. Tudor Hart's observations about hypertension in primary care would serve as an example of a condition falling into this zone.

The doctor and patient engaged in a consultation are themselves complex adaptive systems. They have their own history which influences their current state and they interact with their environment. The time dimension, and interactions within the system and with the environment are crucial to understanding the development of complex adaptive systems. This idea has a close parallel with patient narratives.[3,18] I suggest a new intellectual model is needed that weaves together these three strands:

- the appropriate application of a scientific (probabilistic/linear) method
- the various narratives that make up the patient's health and illness story
- the unpredictable, intuitive, emergent phenomena that emerge in the consultation.

The consultation is the central activity of general practice. The patient's problems, hopes, fears and expectations are explored and the clinician formulates a biomedical diagnosis during the consultation. An exploration of how complexity theory may be applied to this interaction and lead to the development of a new intellectual model of the consultation is described below.

Complexity and a consultation with Mrs Smith

Mrs Jean Smith is a 48-year-old housewife and mother of two late-teenage children. Jean is an alcoholic who works in a local supermarket. She recently faced disciplinary action for drunkenness at work and poor attendance. At home she is unhappy and has suffered alleged sexual abuse from her husband and physical abuse from both her children. She is a heavy smoker with frequent winter chest infections and is being treated for hypertension. She has just been discharged from hospital after a serious suicide attempt. She attended the surgery for a sick-note to return to work. Despite her recent admission to hospital she looked remarkably well, smiling and chatting. She told me how friendly and supportive her family, friends and employer had all been and insisted that she was now ready to turn over a new leaf. Over the past few years I seem to have had little or no impact on this lady's health as I have struggled to get her to face up to her various problems and modify her behaviour to improve her health. Suddenly I had my 'flash' of understanding[4] and I was able to see her as she saw herself – a helpless victim of her circumstances rather than a 'heart-sink' collection of medical diagnostic labels and Read codes.* My sudden insight changed my view of her so that I could see and understand her as she saw herself. I seemed, at last, to have a grasp of her story.

How could complexity theory help to model this consultation? My flash of understanding of her predicament and the subsequent change in diagnostic label from 'alcoholic' to 'victim' was sudden and unpredictable. This change in direction (bifurcation) led me to consider new influences on her health, both negative (risk factors) and positive (medico-social interventions). The patient's recent response (overdosage) could be understood as a reaction to these influences (emergent behaviour). Her overall state of health could be seen as an attractor, which gives a qualitative representation of her life. The factors that influence her at any moment in time will not be quantifiable and her health at any given time will be unpredictable within the overall behaviour of her health system, although it can be observed over time.

Jean Smith can be seen as part of a complex social system.

---

*http://www.cams.co.uk/readcode.htm or http://www.coding.nhsia.nhs.uk/default.asp

Understanding her problems required a lot more effort than the application of a few diagnostic labels (e.g. alcoholic). My new understanding required the ability to see (model) her relationships and roles within her social network. The support and recognition her actions brought from the local community, family and friends were crucial factors in her rehabilitation and somewhat enhanced status after her overdose. She now has a new status and new relationships within the system and, paradoxically, has probably benefited from her actions. These actions have had non-linear effects on herself, her family and carers. Feedback loops have undoubtedly been triggered by recent events, so she has now reached a new state of 'criticality' within her complex environment.

Complexity theory provides both a framework for modelling my patient's health story and a clue to intuitive reasoning. Perhaps my flash of understanding was the final piece in the jigsaw of developing an accurate mental model that (at last) represented something of the complexity of this woman's overall health influences. This shift in understanding came as a revelation to me and can be seen as the result of complex processes within my own mind as I struggled to develop a mental model for my patient. Such a radical shift in my thinking cannot be explained by linear hypothetico-deductive methods or by the recognition of a 'pattern' of illness. I believe that my new understanding of the patient arose as a result of complex processes within my own 'neural-net' that helped me to understand her illness script and the complex nature of her responses to her situation.

This links back to Neighbour's 'right brain responder' and seems to be the antithesis of a logical, linear, hypothetico-deductive or reductionist approach to clinical problem solving, and to demonstrate the need for an integrated, complex and essentially non-linear reasoning model to supplement the traditional scientific clinical method. I suggest that we need to include an opportunity to consider intuitive/non-linear interactions within the consultation, particularly where the issues are difficult and the illness multifactorial. Complexity theory provides such a framework. This links back to the earlier work of Balint, Berne and Neighbour as they all sought to understand and promote clinician behaviours that could enhance the consultation.

Complexity and clinical knowledge

Complexity theory presents us with a challenge to the way that we perceive scientific knowledge. It also affects the way we think about research, particularly about the application of scientific 'method', where the choice of method influences the types of results. Scientific results need to be interpreted in the light of the methods used rather than generalised in ways that may be inappropriate – either to the situation or to the individual patient. The effects of interventions will also be unpredictable for my individual patient. This closely reflects the experience of many clinicians and has profound implications for the interpretation and application of population-based studies to the individual. Using biomedical evidence in clinical practice is difficult, because evidence from group studies cannot predict outcomes for individuals and is further complicated by the context of the consultation.

Perhaps we need to think in new ways based more on the relationships between individuals rather than on deterministic statistical methods. This has traditionally been the realm of qualitative research, but new statistical methods are now being developed that should increase our understanding of complex systems. This has implications for the way we undertake, interpret and enact research results. Population-based research can never predict how an individual will respond to a medical intervention (the doctor or the drug). An individual lives and interacts within a complex social environment. This too will affect that individual's response to treatment. This is particularly important as we enter the brave new world of clinical governance[9] and the pressures that we will be under to apply an evidence-based approach to individual patients and their problems.

The application of complexity theory provides a framework for incorporating non-linear science into clinical practice. This means we can consider narrative and intuition within a scientific clinical methodology.[3] The world is complex, but organised. Descriptions of the world cannot always be reduced to simple deterministic statements. Complexity provides a framework within which we can study the complex, non-linear stories of our patients and our consultations.

Practising medicine requires interpretive skills – recognising the patterns of symptoms and signs that are the essence of an expert clinical method.[13,14] These methods of knowing have more in common with the social sciences, economics and law than the physical sciences.[16] I believe that we should acknowledge the richness and complexity of the social interaction that sits at the heart of the doctor–patient relationship and move away from measurement and reductionist methods.

How is this relevant to the patient and doctor in everyday clinical practice? I believe that we should extend our clinical method to include non-linear science. Complexity theory provides an intellectual framework for the integration of non-linear science into our clinical method. By adopting this approach, clinicians give themselves an opportunity to understand the full richness and complexity of their patients' lives and illness and to open new options for diagnosis, treatment and understanding. We are now in the position to establish a new model for clinical method that incorporates both the science and art of medicine. This demands that the linear and non-linear parts of the consultation must be given equal value and has major implications for learning and teaching clinical method at all levels in future.[19]

What might such a clinical methods model look like? A simple scheme to represent these ideas is shown below (Box 4.1).

Box 4.1 A new model for clinical method – the art and science of medicine

Linear	Non-linear
Traditional scientific method	The 'art' of medicine
Left brain	Right brain
Logical cognitive model	Intuitive cognitive model
Hypothetico-deductive	Interpretive, contextual
Probabilistic	Unpredictable (within boundaries)
Reductionist	Holistic
Quantitative	Qualitative
Evidence-based	Narrative-based
Good for complicated problems	Good for complex problems

Complimenting the traditional scientific clinical method with new models helps us recognise and deal with the intuitive, non-linear, qualitative aspects of the consultation:

- the appropriate application of a scientific method to medical problems (alcoholism, hypertension, smoker)
- the various narratives that make up the patient's health story (family, sexual and work problems)
- the unpredictable, intuitive, Balint-like flash of understanding (patient as powerless victim, understanding of context).

Looking to the future

We can and should use probabilistic reasoning and an evidence-based approach *when it is appropriate to do so*. To fully appreciate our patients and their health needs, we need to understand and apply a clinical method that incorporates the best scientific evidence but also appreciates the illness narrative and the complexity, including the non-linearity, of the patient's and health professional's experience.

The application of complexity theory is not an argument against evidence-based practice. I believe it is possible to practice evidence-based medicine in a complex, narrative-based world.[3] Applying the best available evidence to support an intervention can complement the crucial medical skills of eliciting and interpreting the patient's story. However, in the real world, the evidence base may only apply to a small proportion of our patients.[12] The application of complexity theory to an understanding of the clinical encounter can enhance our models, interpretation and understanding of the problems our patients present to us. Through this better understanding, we should be able to offer appropriate interventions based on a sound clinical method. McWhinney describes general practice as 'the only profession to define itself in terms of relationships, especially the doctor–patient relationship'.[20] He acknowledges the complexity of (general practice) medicine by promoting an organismic rather than mechanistic metaphor of biology. In other words, we are more than the sum of our parts.

These new ideas have major implications for the way that we

record the consultation. Clinical coding methods tend to be reductionist. Recording a consultation with an 8-year-old asthmatic child and his distraught mother in a 5-digit Read code misses all the detail from the narratives of the patient, his mother and the doctor. Coding systems are important for transferring details of drugs, illnesses and allergies but they cannot capture what actually happens in the consultation. 'Lest we forget, for countless patients it is the telling of their stories that helps make them well.'[18]

The NHS is committed to developing electronic health records for all clinical systems over the next few years.[9] These lifelong electronic health records will need to be able to record and present the full range of complex information that patients present to their health professionals throughout their lives. Consultation records will need to have multidimensional links to related problems, people and interventions longitudinally through time. These electronic records will need to be able to model and display this information in a way that helps the clinician understand the complexity of each case. Simple coding structures and problem lists are by definition reductionist and lead to a loss of colour, context and detail. This is very relevant when considering my alcoholic patient. How could a computer present this lady's health story to me in a better way? Could the computer have helped me to see the situation differently earlier?

In this chapter I suggest bringing the non-linear and narrative elements of our clinical practice into a new model for the clinical encounter. I propose that the traditional Newtonian/Cartesian account of the world is inadequate for explaining the complexity of the relationships between a doctor, his patient and the social system in which they both operate. I suggest that complexity theory may help to bridge the gap between the 'science' (linear) and 'art' (non-linear) of medicine. This offers a new paradigm for the extension of our clinical methods to incorporate the intuitive, non-linear and narrative elements of our patients' lives into a new scientific model of the expert clinical method.

Acknowledgements

I would like to thank John Sanfey, Paul Robinson and Ian Purves for their constructive comments, David Byrne, Frances Griffiths,

Jack Cohen and Paul Cilliers for challenging my own orthodoxy and providing such intellectual stimulation.

References

1   Quoted in Cilliers P (1998) *Complexity and Postmodernism: understanding complex systems.* Routledge, London.

2   McWhinney R (1997) *A Textbook of Family Medicine.* Oxford University Press, Oxford.

3   Greenhalgh T (1999) Narrative based medicine in an evidence based world. *BMJ.* **318**: 323–5.

4   Balint M (1957) *The Doctor, His Patient and The Illness.* Tavistock Publications, London.

5   Berne E (1966) *Games People Play.* Andre Deutsch, London.

6   Byrne PS and Long BEL (1976) *Doctors Talking to Patients.* HMSO, London.

7   Working Party of the Royal College of General Practitioners (1972) *The Future General Practitioner: learning and teaching.* British Medical Association, London.

8   Neighbour R (1987) *The Inner Consultation.* Kluwer Academic Publishers, London.

9   Department of Health (1997) *The New NHS: modern, dependable.* The Stationery Office, London.

10   Sackett DL, Straus SE and Richardson WS *et al.* (2000) *Evidence-Based Medicine.* Churchill Livingstone, Edinburgh.

11   Freedman L (1996) Bayesian statistical methods. *BMJ.* **313**: 569–70.

12   Tudor Hart J (1993) Hypertension guidelines: other diseases complicate management. *BMJ.* **306**: 1337.

13   Bordage G and Lemieux M (1991) Cognitive structures of experts and novices. *Academic Medicine.* **66**: S70–2.

14   Groen GJ and Vimla LP (1985) Medical problem solving: some questionable assumptions. *Medical Education.* **19**: 95–100.

15   Griffiths F (1999) Women's control and choice regarding HRT. *Social Science and Medicine.* **49**: 469–81.

16   Cilliers P (1998) *Complexity and Postmodernism: understanding complex systems.* Routledge, London.

17 Wilson T, Holt T and Greenhalgh T (2001) Complexity and clinical care. *BMJ.* **323**: 685–8.

18 Elwyn G and Gwyn R (1999) Stories we hear and stories we tell: analyzing talk in clinical practice. *BMJ.* **318**: 186–8.

19 Robinson P and Heywood P (2000) What do GPs need to know? The use of knowledge in general practice consultations. *British Journal of General Practice.* **49**: 235.

20 McWhinney IR (1996) The importance of being different. William Pickles Lecture 1996. *British Journal of General Practice.* **46**: 433–6.

CHAPTER FIVE

Complexity in epidemiology and public health

Barry Tennison

Summary

Public health is about health and disease in populations rather than in individuals. One of its fundamental sciences is epidemiology, the study of the distribution of disease by person, place and time. However, public health practice is also about acting: taking action that improves health or reduces disease or its impact. This chapter establishes the relevance for public health and epidemiology of complexity theory and complex adaptive systems; discusses the close connections between public health practice, primary care and health improvement; and suggests a research agenda to elucidate both complexity theory applied to public health and epidemiology, and to formulate, from the theory, useful tools for public health practice in primary care and beyond. The chapter illustrates the relevance of complexity to public health by showing how simple mathematical recurrence relationships can help epidemiologists understand the unpredictable prevalence of some diseases, and considers what features of complexity might apply to healthcare systems.

Relevance of complex adaptive systems to epidemiology and public health

Epidemiology takes a population (or perhaps several interacting populations) as its starting point. It is then concerned with the pattern of disease in that population:

- through variations in *person*, i.e. according to characteristics such as sex, age, genetic make-up, occupation, social and family connections, risk factors
- through variations in *place*, i.e. according to geographical aspects such as the overall spatial pattern of the diseases across the relevant area; the association with other factors such as population density, height above sea level, proximity of rivers, minerals, gases; and human structures such as factories, power stations
- through variations in *time*, i.e. regarded as an evolving disease process with a history of incidence and prevalence in the population, as well as a time evolution in each affected person.

Often the most revealing insights are through a combination of these axes, for example viewing a disease as evolving with different time courses through different subpopulations distinguished by age and geography. Examples could be measles progressing through schools and their children, as well as through groups of adults, parents and others, or the associations of multiple sclerosis[1] or some cancers with age, sex and latitude.

Public health builds on epidemiology by factoring in the actions that societies can and do take to modify the patterns of disease, including prevention, cure and care. Public health is also concerned with the effects of healthcare interventions and systems, and how best to deploy these to maximise health and minimise disease and its consequences.

Given the complicated nature of the known and unknown mechanisms for the initiation and transmission of diseases (infectious and non-infectious), it is no wonder that epidemiologists and public health practitioners have been eclectic in seeking help from approaches used in other disciplines such as history,[2] geography,[3] engineering,[4] and mathematics.[5,6] Public health practice is also eclectic in borrowing from economics and health economics, social science, management and organisation theory, and political science.[7] Conversely, other disciplines show a fascination with disease as something on which they can shed light.[8–10]

Three examples are now given to show some ways in which complexity theory and complex adaptive systems are relevant to disease processes, population-level action against disease and healthcare systems.

Example 1: models of disease

One of the simplest types of disease in populations is one caused by a single infectious agent. It is fascinating that even very pared down and simple models for this exhibit complex and chaotic behaviour. We must not be afraid to simplify drastically: this still sheds light and raises disturbing questions.

The simplest modelling exploits the analogy between:

(a) predator–prey processes: in particular, the dynamics of an isolated population of two species (animal or vegetable), one of which preys on the other, while both reproduce
(b) infectious agent processes: in particular, the dynamics of a single infectious agent in a population of susceptible individuals (it matters little for the simple model whether the infection kills or allows recovery, or whether it confers immunity).

Making extreme simplifying assumptions, including random mixing, the modelling in each case leads to an equation (a recurrence relationship) like:

$$x_{t+1} = \alpha x_t(1-x_t)$$

where t denotes time, in a succession of instants, which might be hours, days, weeks or years; α is a parameter, which varies as explained below; and x_t denotes the value of a variable x at the time t.

In the two exemplar cases above, the interpretation of x_t could be, respectively:

(a) the proportion of the total population (prey plus predator) that is prey (at time t)
(b) the point prevalence of the disease at time t (the proportion of the population that is infected).

This equation comes from the logistic map (or function)[11] and is a simplification of the Volterra–Lotka predator–prey models.[12] For the technically minded, the exact form of the recurrence does not really matter for the qualitative behaviour, since this is the generic form of a function with a non-degenerate extremum near that point.[13]

The value of the parameter α is determined partly by the configuration of the system being modelled, and partly by features such as the effectiveness of the predator at killing prey, and their relative reproduction rates, in case (a); or the virulence of the infectious agent and the host resistance, in case (b). So one would expect these, and the values of α, to be relatively stable over time. However α might alter with time, perhaps due to changes in the external environment (e.g. climate, genetic drift or mutation, the effect of other organisms).

The behaviour of x_t with time t depends very markedly on the value of α.[14,15] For values of α less than 3, x_t settles, as t increases, to an equilibrium value. This corresponds to a stable state of the system being modelled, with a constant ratio of predators to prey, or a constant prevalence of the disease circulating in the population. The equilibrium value of x_t is in fact $(1-(1/\alpha))$.

For values of α approaching 3, two things are noticeable. First, it takes longer (in terms of t) for x_t to settle to its equilibrium value. (See below for the relevance of this to secular trends in epidemiology.) Second, before settling, it oscillates around (above and below) the equilibrium value, rather than approaching it smoothly from one side. These phenomena are easily observed on a spreadsheet simulation of the recurrence relation.[16]

For values of α above 3 but less than about 3.4, x_t reaches, as t increases, a kind of steady state where it alternates between two values. In the systems being modelled, this corresponds to regular switching or oscillation between two different states. For example, this could be from a state with many more prey than predators, leading to decimation of the abundant prey by an increasing population of predators, to a state where predators dominate, but then die of hunger (lack of prey) to regain the original state. We might be seeing this on a two-yearly cycle (if t is in years), although in real life the cycles of infectious diseases do not necessarily correspond to the seasons and years.

For values of α above 3.4 but less than about 3.45, x_t takes longer and longer to settle into the period two oscillation, and for values around 3.42 we notice that before settling to period two, x_t seems to cycle through four values. Sure enough, for values of α a little above 3.45, x_t settles into a pattern where it repeats the same four values (a four-cycle).

This phenomenon, where a single equilibrium changes into a two-cycle and then a four-cycle and so on, is known as period doubling, and it is characteristic of the 'transition to chaos'. And indeed, for values of α above 4, as t increases, x_t dots about randomly, with no pattern at all. This is chaos, and has been extensively studied.[17,18]

How is this reflected in the real world? Epidemiologists are familiar with infectious diseases which, in certain populations at certain times, follow a cyclic pattern, such as arboviral encephalitides, measles[19,20] and pertussis; and others, such as plague, polio or psittacosis that seem to have no pattern, whose incidence may be showing chaotic behaviour.[21] Some diseases, such as stomach cancer[22] or multiple sclerosis,[23] exhibit long-term trends (so-called secular trends) for no apparent reason, and this could be a manifestation of an oscillation with long time periods, or a slow move towards an equilibrium position (as above when α was less than 3). Over long time periods, the value of α is likely to make slow changes, so possibly moving the target of the trend. Therefore, some of the puzzling changes in the incidence and prevalence of diseases could be due to a natural underlying dynamic, rather than have specific causes, such as diet, risky behaviour or health-care interventions.

The point here is not to claim that the logistic equation is a particularly good model for diseases in populations in general. First, it is to point out that even a highly simplified non-linear model exhibits remarkably complicated behaviour,[24] which is similar to some seen in the real world. Second, it is to note that there are some general qualitative properties of certain classes of models (such as period doubling, or smooth but slow trends towards equilibrium) which can be adduced even when the detail is too complicated to model.

Elaborations of the simple logistic situation outlined above have been studied in a variety of ways.[25,26] Some epidemiologists are aware of the relevance of complexity theory for studying diseases and the weaknesses of current approaches.[27–29] However, there do seem to be relatively few applications that apply the basic ideas of complexity theory, such as phase space, attractors and bifurcation.

In summary, even at its most basic level, epidemiology studies systems which have the potential for surprisingly complicated behaviour. This is because the kinds of rules, laws and interactions involved are inherently non-linear. Therefore, some parts of complexity theory have great potential relevance for epidemiology, both theoretical and practical.

Example 2: population-level action against disease

Once we consider taking action against diseases and their consequences, we know from experience that we are in an area where results may not match intentions. If we extrapolate from Example 1 above, we may imagine a population of people with great variation in characteristics, with a wide range of diseases, many of which are manifestations of other organisms in their own fight to survive and thrive. It is not surprising that this assembly may form a complex adaptive system (or dissipative structure far from equilibrium,[30] or a self-organising complex system[31] which were introduced in Chapter 1). The results of actions may then be far from what was intended, both because of the tendency of such systems to react in unexpected ways to change (reflecting underlying attractors, rather than externally imposed targets),[32] and because of the 'butterfly' effect of small causes sometimes giving large effects.

If we try to immunise against an infectious disease, it is no surprise that the infectious agent may change its behaviour or evolve, more or less rapidly, in response. For example, some micro-organisms, such as the common cold virus are resistant to population control by immunisation. In other cases, if immunisation levels fall even slightly below a critical level, the disease may be released from control, as when diphtheria re-emerged against a background of economic decline in eastern Europe[33] or in the periodic upswings of pertussis in the UK[34] when immunisation levels fall.[35] More generally, changes in disease patterns and life expectancy are strongly linked in complex ways to changes in socio-economic conditions.[36]

As we are able to give more care which increases life expectancy, we see a changing pattern of diseases in the ageing population. This tendency is also like altering an external parameter on a complex adaptive system.

Other examples of the complications of good intention abound, such as the use of different kinds of vitamin K.[37] Almost all drugs have undesired adverse side effects, which can be viewed as reactions to a disturbance in one of multitudes of highly linked variables by the complex system of the body. The aggregate of these effects can also be seen to affect population health, as for example where the use of antibiotics leads to the emergence of new or different epidemics, whether through resistant organisms or known ones (e.g. TB) somehow being released from control.

In summary, in the area of population-level action against disease, and for health improvement, we know that we are dealing with complex adaptive systems. Further, we know that actions based on good intentions do not always have the desired results, or even desirable results. We know very little about how these systems work, even in comparison with the epidemiology of individual diseases. Any advance in the theories of complexity and complex adaptive systems could have relevance and application for population-level action to improve health and diminish disease.

Example 3: healthcare systems

Any society above a very primitive level has, *de facto*, a healthcare system, comprising the societal efforts (whether more or less organised and planned) to reduce disease and improve health. Observation across time and place suggests that a number of common features or themes then emerge.

First, there is a classic tension between central control and freedom at the front line of care, driven by monetary, economic, accountability, quality and political factors. This becomes more evident in more complicated and sophisticated societies. Second, a national healthcare system comes to be run as one or more organisations, large or small, which interact with each other. Considering the variety of activities, people and technologies involved, and the complicated relationships between them, it is no surprise that the overall healthcare system can be readily conceived as a complex adaptive system with multiple complex adaptive systems nested within it. Chapters 6 and 7, which deal with healthcare organisations and clinical governance explores these ideas further.

A number of features of complex adaptive systems are particularly familiar to those who study healthcare systems. First, there is the influence of positive feedback, as in the ideas of the economist Brian Arthur.[38,39] In particular, increased provision of healthcare often leads to an increased demand for it. Increasing expenditure on healthcare often evokes pressures for even greater spending. Specialisation drives yet greater specialisation. There is probably a great deal to be learned about healthcare systems through studying and applying this new economics.[40]

Second, healthcare systems and organisations are ideal models for applying the complexity theory of organisations[41,42] and leadership and management.[43] On the whole, healthcare organisations are much more complex than those in the manufacturing or service industries. They are very appropriate testing grounds for some of the general theories and approaches.

Some of the management lessons based on complexity theory are already known in other contexts, for example in knowledge about performance management and quality improvement. When trying to achieve a desired performance (perhaps a benchmark or target, for example a low death rate from a disease or from a healthcare intervention, or a low waiting time for care, or a target level of throughput or productivity), there is a danger, well known to engineers, of overcorrecting in response to what is in fact random (or 'common cause') variation.[44] This can easily exaggerate variations in performance beyond what could be achieved. It is a common effect of the use of league tables, or of targets which are unrelated to the performance that the processes involved are actually capable of achieving.[4] Experience in a variety of fields strongly suggests that what is actually needed is an approach which concentrates on improvement, rather than on reward or punishment.[45] There are a number of tools and approaches available to support this, including control charts, process flowcharting, cause and effect analysis and pareto diagrams.[46,47] Some healthcare organisations are taking this kind of approach,[48,49] and in England and Wales, the Commission for Health Improvement (CHI) is maintaining quality improvement as its primary goal, through analysis of systems and processes.[50,51]

In summary, in the area of healthcare systems we know that we are dealing with highly complex organisations. Lessons from applying the theories of complexity and complex adaptive systems to organisations, management and leadership can be tested (and may be tested severely) by applying them to healthcare systems. It is likely that, given the apparent intractability of some of the problems of healthcare systems, attempts will be made to use any available theories and techniques on them, including those emerging from work on complexity.

Some conclusions from the examples

These examples show some of the wide ranging aspects of complexity theory and complex adaptive systems that are applicable to epidemiology and public health. In particular, even the most straightforward of mathematical models for disease processes, as in Example 1, rapidly yield non-linear recurrence relationships or differential equations. With the developing understanding of the qualitative features of non-linear processes, which has progressed over recent years through structural stability theory,[52] catastrophe theory,[53] chaos theory[54] and complexity, has come some increased insight into epidemiology. But there is still much to be gained.

From the point of view of the theories of complex adaptive systems and complexity, we can see that disease processes and patterns, the results of population interventions, and the attributes of healthcare systems may well exhibit:

- non-linear behaviour
- open system behaviour, far from equilibrium
- unexpected responses to disturbance, reflecting underlying attractors in phase space

- bifurcation
- transition to chaos.

These and other lessons from complexity theory potentially provide a rich source of new insights into health and disease.

Public health, primary care and health improvement

Primary care is central to improving the health of the population. This was particularly acknowledged in the Alma Ata 'Health for All' declaration of 1978 and subsequent WHO policies.[55] A considerable amount of effort to develop appropriate kinds of primary care, in different ways, has continued around the world.

Developing countries

In order to achieve optimal health improvement developing countries usually need to focus on widespread basic disease prevention, health promotion and basic healthcare, rather than spend money (and use other resources) on elaborate technical healthcare. There is a tendency for highly technical care to develop in cities, and to benefit very few of the population.

In the developing world, the public health and primary care agenda mainly concerns:

- fundamentals: water, food, hygiene (especially concerning human waste), freedom from violence and oppression
- maternal and child health: family planning, pregnancy, childhood killer diseases (e.g. diarrhoeal diseases), schooling
- debilitating conditions or diseases with an impact on families, work and the economy: e.g. blindness, physical disability, AIDS
- infectious diseases
- education (appropriate education empowers people to take control of their own health and that of their community), especially of women.

The relevance of the theories of complexity and complex adaptive systems to improving health in the developing world therefore seems to lie in:

- applications to epidemiology and control of infectious diseases
- applications to economics and theories of development
- applications to sociology and politics.

Economically rich countries

In economically rich countries, healthcare systems are usually highly developed, and elaborate or complicated healthcare is more or less widely available. Having achieved this, many countries find themselves facing a funding crisis. Usually, it is hard to control expenditure on more and more elaborate forms of healthcare, which are seen as a 'right', in imitation of what happens in the richest countries (who can spend astonishing amounts of money on healthcare).[56] From the point of view of optimising population health and the impact of the interventions used, the need is to increase the emphasis on the care of common conditions with a high impact on the health of a large proportion of the population and on promotion of health and prevention of disease.[57] Failure to do this seems to lead to widespread health inequalities,[58,59] population dissatisfaction, and the dangers of the appearance and reappearance of new and old health problems, such as tuberculosis,[60] sexually transmitted infections, diphtheria, HIV, neurological conditions and the results of animal health problems such as BSE and foot and mouth disease.

In economically rich countries, the public health and primary care agenda mainly concerns:

- maintaining the fundamentals: water quality, food quality and appropriateness, education in hygiene and health, freedom from violence and oppression
- maternal and child health: family planning, pregnancy, keeping childhood killer diseases at bay
- minimising the impact of disability (sensory and physical disability, learning disability, chronic mental health problems, disabling effects of ageing)

- appropriate healthcare, particularly for diseases with a heavy burden, often heart disease, stroke, cancer
- maximising positive health, through exercise, leisure, employment conditions and social opportunities.

The relevance of the theories of complexity and complex adaptive systems to improving health in economically rich countries therefore seems to lie in:

- applications to epidemiology and control of certain diseases, especially cancer, chronic diseases and those associated with advancing age
- applications to healthcare systems, organisation and management
- applications to economics, sociology and politics.

Research agenda

If we are to capitalise on the increasing understanding of complex adaptive systems, their qualitative features, and methods to influence them, then more work is needed to:

- enable those with topic knowledge in epidemiology, public health and primary care to understand more about complexity theory and its applications
- tease out what parts of complexity thinking is actually applicable to health and healthcare
- feed topics and problems which arise in the study of health and disease into the complexity theory agenda.

This may involve relatively traditional research, action research or simply the application of ideas in practice. Some particular research areas or topics which seem worthwhile are as follows.

1 Time-focused epidemiology from the point of view of non-linear systems rather than, for example, estimation of attributable fractions (e.g. different cancers, effects of screening or other preventive activities), ideally focused on policy questions, rather than aetiology.

2   Descriptive phase space portrayals, identification of attractors, description of bifurcations and other complexity behaviour (such as transition to chaos) in health-related areas.
3   Policy appraisals of different health improvement and health-care policies, in terms of likely effects on the complex system, or aiming to give a menu of actions in response to more or less predictable responses.
4   Exploration (from a complexity point of view) of the optimal ways to achieve quality improvement in healthcare: what interventions increase the potential for and usefulness of self-organisation?
5   More study of healthcare management by complexity methods, and use of healthcare management case studies to elucidate complexity and identify possible tools to enhance management effectiveness.
6   Study, using complexity methods, of natural experiments in progress, such as the introduction of new structures (e.g. primary care organisations in the UK), systems and processes (e.g. clinical governance in the UK).
7   Study, using a complexity approach, of effective and less effective methods of external regulation of healthcare organisations.[61]
8   Descriptive studies, in complexity terms, of long-term natural experiments, e.g.
    - changes in healthcare in the USA, through the introduction of health maintenance organisations, managed care, commercial pressures on the hospital system and regulatory methods and effects
    - changes in healthcare in the UK, resulting from different emphases on market mechanisms or cooperative partnership approaches (and differences in the countries making up the UK)
    - changes in continental Europe, especially in the eastern European countries.

References

1   Kesselring J (ed.) (1997) *Multiple Sclerosis.* Cambridge University Press, Cambridge, pp. 49–53.

2   Rosenberg CE (1992) *Explaining Epidemics.* Cambridge University Press, Cambridge.

3   Ricketts TC *et al.* (eds) (1994) *Geographic Methods for Health Services Research.* University Press of America.

4   Mohammed MA, Cheng KK, Rouse A and Marshall T (2001) Bristol, Shipman and clinical governance: Shewhart's forgotten lessons. *Lancet.* **357**: 463–7.

5   Clayton D and Hills M (1993) *Statistical Models in Epidemiology.* Oxford University Press, Oxford.

6   Renton A, Whitaker L, Ison C *et al.* (1995) Estimating the sexual mixing patterns in the general population from those in people acquiring gonorrhea infection – theoretical foundation and empirical findings. *Journal of Epidemiology and Community Health.* **49**: 205–13.

7   http://www.fphm.org.uk/internetpages/exams_frames.htm (Accessed 14 September 2001).

8   Zeeman EC (1976) Duffing's equation in brain modelling. *Bulletin of the Institute of Mathematics.* **12**: 207–14.

9   Cliff AD and Logan JD (1997) A structural time series approach to forecasting the space-time incidence of infectious diseases: post-war measles elimination programmes in the United States and Iceland. In: MM Fischer and A Getis (eds) *Recent Developments in Spatial Analysis: spatial statistics, behavioural modelling and computational intelligence.* Springer Verlag, Berlin, pp. 101–27.

10 Cliff AD, Haggett P and Smallman-Raynor M (1998) *Deciphering Global Epidemics: analytical approaches to the disease records of world cities, 1888–1912.* Cambridge University Press, Cambridge.

11 Nicolis G (1995) *Introduction to Nonlinear Science.* Cambridge University Press, Cambridge, pp. 180-4.

12 May RM (ed.) (1981) *Theoretical Ecology: principles and applications.* Blackwell Scientific, Oxford, pp. 78, 84–6.

13 Nicolis G (1995) *Introduction to Nonlinear Science.* Cambridge University Press, Cambridge, p. 180.

14 Roughgarden J (1979) *Theory of Population Genetics and Evolutionary Ecology: an introduction.* Collier Macmillan, London, pp. 337, 432–50.

15 Baker GL and Gollub JP (1996) *Chaotic Dynamics: an introduction.* Cambridge University Press, Cambridge, pp. 76–89.

16 http://www.complexityprimarycare.org/chaos_demo.htm (Accessed 28 September 2001).

17 Nicolis G (1995) *Introduction to Nonlinear Science.* Cambridge University Press, Cambridge, pp. 192–6.

18 Baker GL and Gollub JP (1996) *Chaotic Dynamics: an introduction.* Cambridge University Press, Cambridge.

19 May RM (ed.) (1981) *Theoretical Ecology: principles and applications.* Blackwell Scientific, Oxford, p. 325.

20 Cliff A, Haggett P and Smallman-Raynor M (1993) *Measles: an historical geography of a major human viral disease from global expansion to local retreat 1840–1990.* Blackwell, Oxford, pp. 305–34.

21 http://www.cdc.gov/mmwr/preview/mmwrhtml/mm4853a1.htm (Part 2) (Accessed 14 September 2001).

22 http://www.doh.gov.uk/hpsss/tbl_a3.htm (Accessed 13 September 2001).

23 Sumelahti M-L, Tienari PJ, Wikström J *et al.* (2001) Increasing prevalence of multiple sclerosis in Finland. *Acta Neurologica Scandinavica.* **103**: 153–8.

24 May R (1976) Simple mathematical models with very complicated dynamics. *Nature.* **261**: 459–67.

25 Kendall BE and Fox GA (1998) Spatial structure, environmental heterogeneity, and population dynamics: analysis of the coupled logistic map. *Theoretical Population Biology.* **54**: 11–37.

26 Schuster HG (1995) *Deterministic Chaos: an introduction.* Weinheim, Cambridge.

27 Phillippe P and Mansi O (1998). Nonlinearity in the epidemiology of complex health and disease processes. *Theoretical Medicine and Bioethics.* **19**: 591–607.

28 Bloom LA and Bloom BS (1999) Decision analytic modeling in health care decision making. Oversimplifying a complex world? *International Journal of Technology Assessment in Health Care.* **15**: 332–9.

29 Earn DJ, Rohani P, Bolker BM and Grenfell BT (2000) A simple model for complex dynamical transitions in epidemics. *Science.* **287**: 667-70.

30 Capra F (1996) *The Web of Life.* HarperCollins, London, pp. 172–8.

31 Kauffman S (1993) *The Origins of Order.* Oxford University Press, Oxford, pp. 21–5.

32 Nokes DJ and Anderson RM (1987) Rubella vaccination policy: a note of caution. *Lancet.* **20**: 1441–2.

33 http://www.phls.co.uk/facts/immunisation/diphtheria/diptintro.htm (Accessed 14 September 2001).

34 http://www.phls.co.uk/facts/immunisation/whooping%20cough/whonotdth graph.htm (Accessed 14 September 2001).

35 Gangarosa EJ, Galazka AM, Wolfe CR *et al.* (1998) Impact of the anti-vaccine movements on pertussis control: the untold story. *Lancet.* **351**: 356–61.

36 Chenet L, McKee M, Fulop N *et al.* (1996) Changing life expectancy in central Europe: is there a single reason? *Journal of Public Health Medicine.* **18**: 329–36.

37 Tripp JH and McNinch AW (1998) The vitamin K debacle: cut the Gordian knot but first do no harm. *Archives of Diseases in Childhood.* **79**: 295–7.

38 Arthur WB (1990) Positive feedbacks in the economy. *Scientific American.* **February**: 80–5.

39 Arthur WB (1994) *Increasing Returns and Path Dependence in the Economy.* University of Michigan Press, Ann Arbor.

40 Waldrop MM (1994) *Complexity: the emerging science at the edge of order and chaos.* Penguin, Harmondsworth.

41 Battram A (1998) *Navigating Complexity.* The Industrial Society, London.

42 Mitleton-Kelly E (1998) *Organisations As Complex Evolving Systems.* http://www.lse.ac.uk/lse/complex/pdfiles/publication/organisation_as_complex_evolving_systems.pdf (Accessed 7 September 2001).

43 Wheatley M (2000) *Leadership and the New Science.* Berrett-Koehler Publishers, San Francisco, CA.

44 Oakland JS (1996) *Statistical Process Control.* Butterworth-Heinemann, Oxford, pp. 63–72.

45 Berwick DM (1996) A primer on leading the improvement of systems. *BMJ.* **312**: 619–22.

46 Oakland JS (1996) *Statistical Process Control.* Butterworth-Heinemann, Oxford.

47 Montgomery DC (1996) *Introduction to Statistical Quality Control.* John Wiley & Sons, New York.

48 James B (2001) *Understanding Variation: Statistical Process Control (SPC).* http://www.ihc.com/institute/8.3/8.3.presentationfiles/8.3.4.variation.pdf (Accessed 12 September 2001).

49 Benneyan JC (1998) Statistical quality control methods in infection control and hospital epidemiology, part I: introduction and basic theory. *Infection Control and Hospital Epidemiology.* **19**: 194–214.

50 http://www.chi.nhs.uk/eng/cgr/whatis.shtml (Accessed 14 September 2001).

51 James B (2001) *Managing Clinical Processes: Doing Well by Doing Good.* http://www.ihc.com/institute/8.3/8.3.presentationfiles/8.3.2.methods.pdf (Accessed 12 September 2001).

52 Thom R (1972) *Stabilité Structurelle et Morphogénèse.* Benjamin, New York.

53   Zeeman EC (1977) *Catastrophe Theory*. Addison-Wesley, London.

54   Baker GL and Gollub JP (1996) *Chaotic Dynamics: an introduction*. Cambridge University Press, Cambridge.

55   http://www.who.int/inf-pr-1998/en/pr98-89.html (Accessed 14 September 2001).

56   http://www.oecd.org/els/health/software/table9.xls (Accessed 14 September 2001).

57   Rose G (1992) *The Strategy of Preventive Medicine*. Oxford University Press, Oxford.

58   Government Statistical Service (1997) *Health Inequalities Decennial Supplement*. The Stationery Office, London.

59   http://www.doh.gov.uk/healthinequalities/index.htm (Accessed 14 September 2001).

60   Rose AM and Watson JM *et al.* (2001) Tuberculosis at the end of the 20th century in England and Wales: results of a national survey in 1998. *Thorax.* **56**: 173–9.

61   Walshe K (1999) Improvement through inspection? The development of the new Commission for Health Improvement in England and Wales. *Quality in Healthcare.* **8**: 191–201.

Introduction

There is something not quite right with health service planning and delivery. Research has little direct influence on health service policy,[1] organisational change has little effect on service provision,[2] rational priority setting frameworks remain elusive,[3] and health economists continue to develop technical solutions that have no impact at grassroots level.[4,5] At an administrative level, decision makers demonstrate a predilection for process rather than outcome indicators[6] and the picture is often one of 'organisations under siege, barely coping' where managers present 'glossy corporate images that belie the problems of working in organisations as complex as the NHS'.[7] At a service provision level, complementary therapy challenges the popularity of mainstream medicine in the absence of any evidence base,[8] general practitioners (GPs) seem reluctant to follow evidence-based guidelines[9] but implement small changes that they consider an improvement on current systems,[10] and 'street bureaucrats' develop pragmatic coping strategies that allow them to process citizens through the system.[11]

Against this background, demographic, epidemiological and socio-economic developments are driving demands for improvements in the efficiency and quality of healthcare delivery. As a result of this pressure, healthcare systems across the world are experiencing a series of policy dilemmas that have been identified as a series of five shifts.[12]

- When is care delivered? – the balance between prevention and treatment.
- Where is it delivered? – the balance between institutional and community care.
- How is it delivered? – the balance between patient and professional involvement in care.
- What is delivered? – the balance between knowledge and habit-based care.
- Who is cared for? – the need to balance care equitably between different sections of society.

These tensions have resulted in a search for new ways of realigning healthcare organisations reflecting a broader agenda to modernise and improve public services as a whole. However, no model has emerged as the right answer and health systems across the world have yet to adopt similar organisational themes.

This chapter will set the search for policy instruments in a historical perspective before considering how insights from complex adaptive systems theory might be applied to NHS policy formulation and delivery. It does not aim to offer an exhaustive review of the area (a useful bibliography is given by Plsek[13] – www.ihi.org/iomreport/10M2.htm) or compare complexity thinking with other methods of managing organisational change (a comprehensive review is given by Iles[14] – www.sdo.lshtm.ac.uk).

The development of healthcare policy – the road to post-normal healthcare

To illustrate the evolution of healthcare delivery, a framework proposed by Ouchi[15] is developed as shown in Figure 6.1. This approach shows the mode of operation of the health service related to how well the transfer process, which relates inputs (resources) to outputs (health), is understood and how well outputs can be defined. The historical stages are as follows.

- *The first way* Managerial command: a focus on hierarchy and control.
- *The second way* The purchaser–provider split: developing market forces.
- *The third way* Integrating cooperation and competition: attempting to get the best of both worlds.
- *The fourth way* Understanding the health service as a complex adaptive system: post-normal healthcare.

The first way: managerial command and control

There was little in the way of formal management for the first 25 years of the NHS and the focus was on the centrality of clinical freedom. Management was perceived as diplomacy, in which every effort was made to reach an accommodation between interested parties in matters of a sensitive or controversial nature.[16]

In the early 1980s, a fundamental shift took place that reflected

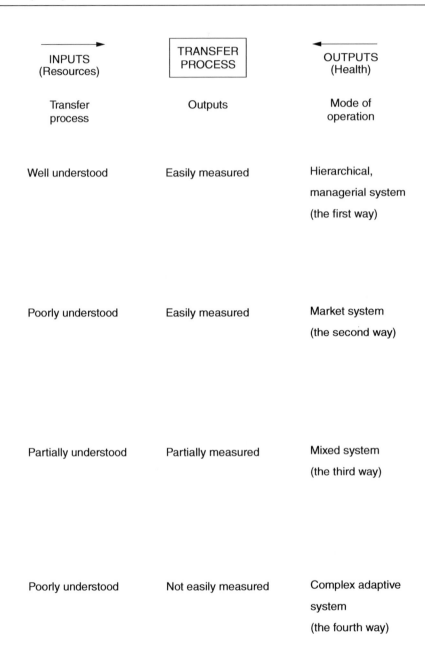

Figure 6.1 Four models of health systems depending on how well the transfer process that relates inputs (resources) to outputs (health) is understood and how well outputs can be defined.

government interest in more systematic approaches to public service organisation. In the healthcare sector, the Griffiths enquiry was directed to examine ways in which NHS resources were controlled, with the aim of securing the best value for money. The report highlighted the lack of managerial accountability and was critical of the system of consensus management. As Griffiths wrote 'if Florence Nightingale were carrying her lamp through the corridors of the NHS today, she would almost certainly be searching for the people in charge'.[17]

Over the prevailing years, a hierarchical managerial approach was consolidated that focused on objectives, performance and accountability. The dominant metaphor of policy analysis and implementation was the machine – each part of the health service had a predefined function contributing to the overall purpose with government pulling the levers.

The second way: from hierarchies to markets

When it is perceived that the transfer process between inputs and outputs is poorly understood but that outputs are readily measured, Ouchi's model suggests that a market approach may be the best framework within which to distribute resources. However, during the late 1980s there were more practical concerns. A number of financial crises instigated a wide-ranging review of the NHS that was conducted largely in secret. The problem was seen to be inefficiency produced by entrenched professionals and administrators operating in an environment of perverse incentives with no impetus for change. Influenced by a small number of health economists, and finding spiritual support from the market tendencies of the Thatcher government, the White Paper *Working for Patients*[18] outlined a radical agenda.

The main features of reform were the separation of purchaser from provider function and the development of GP fundholding within a quasi-market for health. This highly politicised atmosphere split professional allegiances, bewildered the public and caused considerable managerial conflict. In fact, the implementation of managed competition required more rules and regulations than the system that preceded it and overall, despite some changes in culture, measurable changes were small.[19]

By the end of the 1990s a political consensus was to develop that acknowledged that the essential features of the reforms were worth keeping. However, the metaphor of a market place where goods and services are bought and sold in an environment of low trust and low cooperation was to be replaced by a system that sought to balance the advantages of the first and second ways. Box 6.1 shows the problems that this new approach attempted to overcome.

Box 6.1 Some problems with the machine or market approaches

- Machines are static and respond only to what they are designed to do – power is invested in the designer.
- Market power accrues to the larger players with more resources.
- Machines or markets cannot encompass competing goals or objectives.
- The interdependency and connectivity between elements of the system cannot be accommodated by machines or markets – the importance of enduring relationships and informal networks is overlooked.
- The problems of public sector management are often highly context-dependent requiring specific solutions for specific situations.

The third way: integrating cooperation and competition

The new approach to NHS organisation was known as 'the third way' in healthcare reform. The theoretical framework had been developed in the mid-1990s by Giddens[20] who argued that rigid hierarchical state structures were increasingly incapable of fulfilling the diverse needs of citizens, and markets alone would not provide economic success or acceptable social outcomes. The third way advocated a mixed economy that promoted a synergy between public and private sectors, utilising the dynamics of markets but with the public interest in mind. This pragmatic approach to public policy reform was reflected in the government White Paper – *The New NHS: modern, dependable.*[21] The aim was to retain the elements of the purchaser–provider split but emphasise a more collaborative approach with longer-term arrangements.

The third way demanded some difficult balancing acts, for example between central direction or local autonomy, or between the use of sanctions or incentives to direct behaviour. This search for a middle path has resulted in a cocktail of organisations and directives issued under the guise of a 'modernisation agenda'. One interpretation is that by making use of a variety of instruments ministers will increase their chances of getting something right!

Although the third way seeks to define a balance between market and managerial approaches (Box 6.2), the focus remains on top-down analysis and control, overlooking the fact that healthcare issues are multidimensional, complex and contingent, and take place against a background of limited room for manoeuvre for managers and practitioners. What has made the third way so difficult to achieve in practice and attract so much theoretical criticism is its failure to recognise its partial shift to a complexity-based frame of reference – the fourth way.

Box 6.2 Elements of the third way – a question of balance

- Striking a balance between central direction and local autonomy.
- The recognition of competition as a lever to efficient use of resources.
- An emphasis on longer-term cooperation.
- A shift to a private sector management style away from a public service ethic.
- An emphasis on performance and output measurement.
- An emphasis on patient involvement and empowerment.
- An emphasis on national frameworks of care with subsequent monitoring.

The fourth way: recognising the NHS as a complex adaptive system

Although the machine model has been effective as a means of generating economic development in conditions of simple modernisation, this approach becomes less applicable as societies and economies become more complicated and reflexive. Systems thinking grew out of the observations that there were many phenomena that modern scientific analysis could not explore due to positive and negative feedback between elements of an organisation.

A system is a set of connected elements that have a defined purpose but which demonstrate properties of the whole rather than the constituent parts.[22] The fourth way or post-normal healthcare views the NHS as a hierarchy of interrelated systems that interact in a non-linear fashion. The emphasis moves away from a linear analysis leading to prediction and control to an appreciation of the configuration of relationships and an understanding of what creates patterns of order and behaviour among a system's components. The important features are connectivity, recursive feedback, and the existence of self-ordering rules that give systems the capacity to emerge as new patterns of order.

The development of chaos theory offers new mathematical insights into the properties of non-linear systems but equations that define interactions between variables remain unchanged. However, in human systems, these algorithms or mental models are continually changing as agents adapt and co-evolve with their environment. Because of this, a quantitative approach to non-linear interaction in human systems is limited and complexity draws upon the metaphors of chaos to obtain qualitative insights into organisational behaviour. Four metaphors are important when considering healthcare organisation: mental models, phase space, attractors, and simple rules.

Mental models

Agents operate according to their own internal rules or mental models for how they respond to the environment. Because agents can both change and share their internal rules, complex systems can learn and adapt over time. Complexity is the result of the rich non-linear interaction of agents' mental models in response to the local information they are presented with.

Phase space and attractors

Complex systems can be described using the metaphor of a multidimensional phase space. Each system variable is defined and quantified in one dimension. Agents will follow trajectories through this space with time but, although their path cannot be predicted with certainty, attractors place limits on their room for manoeuvre. For example, in a system such as a general practice, attractors could be maximisation of income or rapid access to health care provision. Attractors in the UK health system are equity and efficiency. In the USA profit is a powerful attractor. Organisational attractors emerge from the interaction of mental models, usually over a relatively long period of time.

As information can be distributed across the whole of phase space and interaction is invariably non-linear, small changes in one area of phase space can have large effects across the whole system. For example, the riding accident of the actor Christopher Reeves had a large but probably inappropriate impact on the redistribution of research funding into spinal injuries in the USA.[23] Alternatively, large influences may result in negligible outcomes. *The Health of the Nation* initiative was a major strategic NHS initiative designed to influence health but a retrospective analysis confirmed it as a failure with little impact on the targets it sought to influence.[24]

Simple rules

One approach that is finding practical relevance is the contention that the recursive application of relatively simple rules or guiding principles *applied locally* can lead to complex, emergent and innovative system behaviour. The suggestion is that systems often organise themselves around a limited number of simple rules or guiding principles that may remain at the subconscious level. One way of looking at simple rules is as fundamentals of mental models that are shared by members of an organisation. Bringing these rules into a level of awareness offers the opportunity to investigate their implications and change them. By identifying the underlying rules of a system and changing them where relevant, the system may emerge in a more desirable pattern of order.

Plsek identifies three types of simple rules for human systems:[13]

- general direction pointing
- system prohibition, i.e. setting boundaries
- resource or permission providing.

He suggests that simple rules and experimentation on a small scale will drive the emergent behaviour of a health system to a desired pattern.

Box 6.3 An example of some simple rules for the development of healthcare[25]

- Accept that death, sickness and pain are part of life.
- Medicine has limited powers, particularly to solve social problems, and is risky.
- Doctors don't know everything – they need decision-making and psychological support.
- We are all in this together.
- Patients can't leave problems to doctors.
- Doctors should be open about their limitations.
- Politicians should refrain from extravagant promises and concentrate on reality.

Simple rules can be discovered through the use of narrative or observation and have found favour as a practical framework in which complexity insights can be utilised. However, they have been criticised in a number of areas. A major concern is that this approach reflects the ideology of control that the complexity framework seeks to avoid and fails to address the subtleties of human interaction.

The interpretation and application of these insights to healthcare organisation remains contested. Here, I suggest that the metaphors of complexity be used as a pragmatic toolkit – using them when they seem to be useful, returning them to the shelf when they are not.

Healthcare organisation and culture

At a general level, organisations exist to enable people to accomplish the joint action required for human living.[26] Recent attempts to instigate change in the NHS have invoked the notion of changing the organisation and its culture.[27] But what is an organisation and how is its culture identified?

What is an organisation?

The traditional view reflects the machine metaphor. Organisations have set objectives, fixed interactions, defined boundaries and operate under a hierarchical power structure. Fraser[28] identifies the need for a degree of structure for areas such as finance and governance but stresses that boundaries should be flexible and permeable. The focus is on the boundaries between individuals and not organisations, creating space to develop enabling connections and interactions, removing controls and embracing surprise. Power is seen as the capacity to act generated by relationships underpinned by clear purpose. Stacey[26] develops this theme and argues that organisations can never possess identity because they are not things but processes, continually responding and potentially transformed. He focuses on the central role of ordinary everyday conversation between people at a local level from which meaning or knowledge emerges within the conflicting restraints of power relationships. Organisational identity emerges through the process of relating.

An alternative perspective is to view organisations as areas of phase space that share local attractors. Boundaries are indistinct but characterised by a diminution of information flow. Agents within an organisation send out projections to other subspaces and are aware of projections from them. Through time their trajectories will take them into other areas of phase space. For example, while at work as a GP, my local attractor is patient health; I go home where the attractor changes to family security; in the evening, I visit my vintage car club where the attractor is the preservation of vintage cars.

Organisational culture

The concept of organisational culture arose in the management literature of the 1980s and represents the values, norms and patterns of action that characterise social relationships within a formal organisation.[29] Attempts at cultural change have viewed organisations as concrete entities with variables that can be isolated, described and manipulated. However, healthcare organisations are different in many respects from other sectors where cultural change has been instigated. For example, stakeholders have disparate schemes of values and beliefs and there is domination by strong professions who not only have the power to constrain change but have a unique relationship with service users. Davies[30] has described the contested nature of health service culture. Highlighting the lack of research in the area he presents a sober assessment of the task of cultural transformation in this sector.

Box 6.4 The elements of organisational culture (from Davies[30])

- Assumptions – the 'taken for granted' views of the world, e.g. medical research predicated on the use of modern science and the feasibility of transferring knowledge.
- Values – the basic foundations for making judgements and distinguishing right from wrong, e.g. putting the needs of the patient first above broader societal objectives.
- Artefacts – the physical and behavioural manifestations of culture, e.g. dress codes, peer review, secondary care consultant 'firms'.

Does shifting to a complexity frame of reference offer new insights into the nature of culture and its place within an organisation? Assumptions, values and artefacts could reflect the simple rules that direct the interaction between people at a local level and that affect the meaning of their lives. For example, three cultures within a primary care organisation can be identified by their simple rules as follows:

- *healthcare professionals* – do what is best for the patient, base decisions on quantitative evidence where possible
- *social care professionals* – act in the interests of the community, reflect legislative frameworks, are suspicious of quantitative evidence
- *managers* – define objectives, monitor performance, respond to authority.

The attractors for the environment in which they operate could be maximisation of the welfare of the population, including considerations of equity and efficiency. But can these insights help to manage change?

Changing the organisation

From description to prescription in healthcare systems

Models help us to see pattern in the world around us and interpret events in terms of that perceived pattern. We create reality, rather than observe it, around 'bundles of related assumptions', conceptual lenses through which we view the world. Models help us with four basic questions:

1 What does happen?
2 What will happen?
3 What would we like to happen? (For this stage, objectives need to be defined and values made explicit so that judgements can be made about what is right or wrong.)
4 How can we make it happen using insights from the model?

Since the time of the Enlightenment, the predominant model for science has been the machine. Outcomes are predictable and systems can be understood by breaking them down into their component parts. Complex systems are seen to need complex rules to understand them and when these do not yield the required results, even more rules are created. Approximations and statistical manipulations are used to adjust for discrepancies while predictive limitations are seen to reflect inadequacies, omissions, bias or randomness.

Within the context of healthcare, the objective is to improve the health of the nation and is underpinned by the values of efficiency and equity. Professional activity consists of instrumental problem solving by the rigorous application of scientific theory and techniques, which involve the application of general principles to specific problems. Implicit resource decisions undertaken by clinicians are seen as incoherent and lead to inefficiency and inequity.[31]

Box 6.5 Elements of the 'modern' approach to problems in healthcare

- Linear – there is a simple relationship between inputs and outputs; small inputs have small effects, large inputs have large effects.
- Deterministic – the future of a system can be predicted with certainty.
- Reductionist – systems can be understood by breaking them down into their component parts.
- Analytical – the system can be understood and engineered towards defined objectives.
- Impartiality – an observer can stand outside the system without being influenced by it.

The success of modern science is indisputable. However, arising initially from concerns in the field of quantum physics and more recently from the development of non-linear systems theory, the application of this simplistic world view to many systems has been questioned. In organisations, Stacey[26] identifies three areas of analytical approach depending on the certainty about how outputs are related to inputs and on agreement about this certainty (*see* Figure 6.2).

When there is a high degree of certainty about outcomes from actions and of agreement amongst the agents involved in the actions, machine systems thinking with detailed planning and control is appropriate. This 'rational decision-making' framework

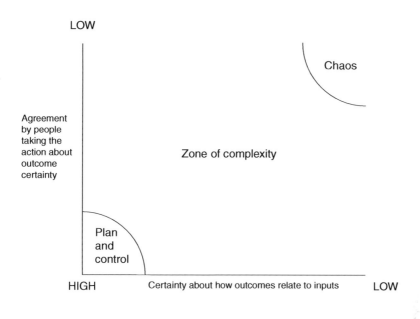

Figure 6.2 The Stacey diagram (chaos is used in its lay interpretation).

involves defining and ranking values, specifying objectives, identifying relevant options, calculating the consequences and costs of these options, and choosing the option that maximises the defined values.

The 'garbage can model' sits at the other end of the spectrum and is the antithesis of the rational approach. It sees organisations as a continual mixture of people, choices and problems circulating aimlessly and occasionally coinciding to create a juncture at which a decision is made – a collection of choices looking for problems, solutions looking for the issues to which they might be the answer and decision makers looking for work.[32]

The zone between these extremes has been described in policy terms as disjointed incrementalism or 'muddling through'. In this zone decisions are seen as incremental, experimental and 'satisficing' – accommodating, satisfying and sufficing behaviour.[33] Complexity theory offers us new insights into how this zone operates.

When applying Stacey's model to organisational management, the trick is to match the approach with the complexity of the task. A rational approach underpinned by the principles of modern science is important in areas where there is likely to be a high degree of predictability. For example, a linear approach is clearly preferable when undertaking tasks such as cardiac resuscitation, a hip replacement operation, or building a new hospital. However, much of health service organisational activity takes place where there is uncertainty over how outputs can be measured and over the nature of the transfer process that converts inputs to outputs. Viewing the process, known as disjointed incrementalism or muddling through, as a complex one offers new possibilities for health service management and development.

Changing complex systems

Complexity theory can facilitate an understanding of what creates patterns of order and behaviour, offering useful descriptive insights. But can it be used to manage cultural and organisational change in the required direction? The answer is contested and within the field of complexity there is a spectrum of opinion.

On the left wing of the debate, it is argued that we can never move further than a descriptive picture. Organisational life is seen as a 'complex responsive process' and focuses on the emergence of radically unpredictable aspects of complex systems. The future cannot be predicted or influenced but is being continually created by the interactions of agents in the present. This occurs predominately outside an organisation's legitimate systems of hierarchy, rules and communication patterns, within the 'shadow organisation' that lies behind the scenes (e.g. hallway conversations).[26]

On the right wing is the systems approach – a belief that complex systems are objective realities outside of which policy makers can stand and control towards desired end points using insights derived from complexity science. For example, Miller[34] identifies three strategies that can be applied to health systems.

- Joining recognises and enhances existing attractors. For example, the attractor of a patient's desire to stop smoking will be enhanced when associated with the attractor of pregnancy.
- Transforming seeks to change an attractor or create a new one. This can either be done by 'wedging' where small positive changes push the system towards the desired attractor, by

increasing information flow, or by increasing connections between agents in a particular manner.

- Hammering involves externally changing an attractor through intentional coercion. For example, the imposition by government of the purchaser–provider split in the NHS.

To the centre-right is an approach that calls for the redesign of healthcare systems from within. The emphasis is on identifying simple rules and management prescriptions drawn from complexity insights.[35] Some of these principles are shown in Box 6.6.

Box 6.6 Some principles for managing complex adaptive systems[36]

- Good enough vision – provide minimum specifications, rather than try to plan out every detail.
- Clockwear/swarmwear – balance data and intuition, planning and acting, safety and risk.
- Tune to the edge – foster the right degree of information flow, connectivity, diversity and difference instead of controlling information, forcing agreement and working sequentially.
- Shadow system – listen to the shadow system and recognise its importance to the two agents' mental models and subsequent actions.
- Chunking – allow complex systems to emerge out of the links among simple systems that work well and are capable of operating independently.
- Paradox – uncover and use paradox rather than avoiding it as if it was unnatural.

The left of centre sees learning as the strategy for cultural change. This approach acknowledges that the future is not always predictable but boundable and that taking action and seeing what happens is often the best we can do. Learning organisations use knowledge to develop structures and human resources that are flexible, adaptable and responsive.[37,38] By encouraging rich, diverse and dynamic relationships, new sets of interactions emerge that form solutions that are not necessarily optimal but nevertheless satisfactory for the constraints put on the system. Three types of learning have been recognised:[39]

- Single loop learning leads to incremental improvements to existing practice, i.e. maintaining a steady direction through the use of a feedback loop. Single loop learning tends to leave organisational objectives largely unchanged, e.g. clinical audit where existing practice is compared with explicit standards.
- Double loop learning occurs when organisations rethink basic goals, norms, and paradigms, i.e. they reflect upon their simple rules, mental models and attractors.
- Meta-learning reflects an organisation's attempts to learn about and improve its ability to learn.

In the NHS, the Modernisation Agency has adopted a form of single loop learning based on a rapid cycle 'plan-do-study-act' methodology and the development of collaboratives to share good practice.[40] However, true learning organisations have a number of more fundamental characteristics that include flat hierarchical structures, an emphasis on teamwork, individual empowerment, information sharing, openness, creativity, experimentation, an ability to risk failure and learn from mistakes. There is encouragement to move beyond traditional professional or departmental boundaries, changing the way people conceptualise issues and allowing for new creative approaches to old problems.

Developing learning organisations may offer the best option for change. In the complex environment of the health service we must educate not merely for competence (what individuals know and are able to do in terms of knowledge, skills and attitude), but for capability (the ability to change, generate new knowledge and continuously improve performance). Health service leadership changes from transactional to transformational. A transactional leader has a strong sense of direction and comes to an agreement with subordinates about what each will do to make a reality of a given vision. A transformational leader is at the centre of a socially constructed network allowing a vision to emerge from interaction and dialogue. The focus shifts to an emphasis on process, supporting learners rather than defining goals with rigid and prescriptive content.[41] Underpinning this concept is an appreciation of the importance of social capital.

Developing social capital in organisations

Organisations utilise three forms of capital – physical, human and social.[42] Physical capital consists of the material resources that make up the health service. Human capital comprises the endowment of education, information and knowledge within the workforce. Social capital reflects the interaction based on social and professional networks. Within the context of learning systems, human capital and social capital comprise distributed intelligence – adapting and co-evolving with the environment and each other, learning what works and what does not. This model sees the practitioners embedded in a network of other professionals delivering team-based care and showing the attributes of openness and repricocity in an atmosphere of shared information and shared learning.

Inevitably there must be a balance between checking and trusting but in the absence of trust and mutual obligation, staff retreat to an environment of mistrust and self-preservation within a context of organisational decline.[43] Box 6.7 identifies some characteristics of high and low trust relations.

Box 6.7 Characteristics of high and low trust relations (from Fox[44])

High trust
- Share ends and values.
- Have a diffuse sense of long-term obligation.
- Offer support without calculating the cost or expecting an immediate return.
- Communicate freely and openly with each other.
- Be prepared to risk their fortunes in the others' party.
- Give the benefit of doubt in relation to motives and goodwill if there are problems.

Low trust
- Have divergent goals and interests.
- Have explicit expectations which must be reciprocated through balanced exchanges.
- Carefully calculate the costs and benefits of any concessions.

- Restrict and screen communications in their own separate interests.
- Attempt to minimise their dependence on others' discretion.
- Are suspicious about mistakes or failures.

In summary, to improve healthcare we need not better professionals but better systems of work where the trick is to attend more to the interaction than to the elements.[45] A useful first step would be to understand the importance of learning and the nature of social capital that holds organisations together, underpinned by the concept of trust.

Changing the policy metaphor – from health service engineer to health systems gardener

Viewing the NHS as an ecosystem[46] can offer useful insights into organisational delivery. Each agent cannot be understood in isolation. All parts adapt by learning to survive in a topography that is provided by coexisting and changing parts. Ecosystems cannot be engineered – there are no causal links that promise sophisticated tools for analysing and predicting system behaviour. However, they can be nurtured.

Unfortunately, policy makers remain trapped in the 'modern' approach – a view that an independent observer can stand outside the system and engineer it towards desired goals. Implicit decisions undertaken by practitioners and managers are seen as incoherent leading to inefficiency and inequity.[31] This policy framework dictates that complex systems require explicit, technical rules and when these do not yield the required results, the answer is to create even more rules.

Foucault[47] has described the concept of governmentality. This recognises a move away from government as a 'master institution'[48] – a dominant status that lies outside the citizenry, setting objectives and directing policy. The emphasis becomes one of managing and overseeing a population so that they flourish. The focus is on the 'conduct of conduct' – the shaping and guiding of people so that they do what is best for themselves and society as a whole. This approach moves government to the role of gardener, facilitating rich interaction within the system from which satisfactory solutions will emerge. The emphasis is on encouragement to explore the system's environment, sharing feedback and clearing pathways but always within defined boundaries.

There is a more fundamental need for government to stand partially outside the system. Funtowicz[49] draws a distinction between *ordinary complexity* and *emergent complexity*. Ordinary complexity is characterised by a complimentarity of competition and cooperation within a diversity of elements and subelements. Stability and simple system goals are the main features. Emergent complexity, in contrast, frequently oscillates between hegemony (the predominance of one element over all others) and fragmentation as diversity and innovation are impeded. The hegemonies of the NHS are well recognised. Precedence, tradition and vested interests still remain.[50] Governmentality guards against emergent complexity – providing of course there is a rich interaction between government and citizens.

Implications for health service research in complex healthcare organisations

The need to make evidence-based decisions has permeated all areas of public policy and healthcare is no exception. Against a background of increasing demands on limited resources, the emphasis is on providing healthcare based on evidence of effectiveness (does it work?) and cost-effectiveness (is it worth paying for?). Black[1] has warned of the implicit assumption of a linear relation between research evidence and policy and suggests that researchers should be cautious about uncritically accepting the notion of evidence-based policy. The problems of obtaining evidence to inform service development are recognised and include:[51]

- the danger of asserting the hegemony of a particular type of evidence
- the problem of different timetables of research and policy making

- exaggerated claims over what research can deliver
- the unfeasibility of divorcing the policy processes from current political agendas.

Nevertheless, current wisdom still reflects a reductionist approach to the investigations of even complex systems and a phased evaluation that remains underpinned by the randomised controlled trial.[52] Non-linear interactions between agents are seen as confounding variables in an otherwise perfect study methodology.

It is not enough to know that something works. We need to know if it is worth paying for? Health economics is a subdiscipline of economics that offers a framework relating the benefits of competing interventions to the resources incurred in their production. Building on a small number of axioms, health economists seek to reduce the complex motives and interactions of stakeholders to explicit and rational decision-making frameworks.

At grass-roots level the impact of health economics on decision making has been imperceptible.[53] At a national level, a review of countries that have attempted to tackle the rationing agenda suggests that the process of resource allocation is complex and extremely messy. There has been no convergence towards any explicit framework that is acceptable both publicly and politically.[54] Value judgements, estimates and gut feelings remain the predominant determinates of outcome[55] in an area hedged with constraints, an infinite variety of intermediate positions, arguments and counter arguments.

Butler[56] argues that a sensitive and intelligent kind of muddling through seems to accord with the reality of how resources are allocated at the coal face and argues that the discourses about what is right and what is feasible must keep in step with each other. Hunter has argued that decision making in healthcare is an iterative process embracing patient intervention and cost-effectiveness variables from which a decision is made.[57] However, these commentators fail to set their insights within a complexity frame of reference.

Vernacular health economics needs to be developed to accommodate the insights that health economics has to offer, but recognising the limitations of applying a linear discipline to a non-linear environment.[58] The emphasis is on pragmatism and developing approaches that recognise that most commissioners of healthcare don't want to change the world but seek to make marginal change in a complex system on the basis of historical precedent and limited room for manoeuvre.

Due to the complex nature of healthcare organisations, new research approaches will be needed where research and development is integral to what all managers and practitioners do and which reflects the context in which they operate. Research techniques need to frame problems as well as solve them and decision makers should accept satisfactory rather than optimal solutions. Any research approach must be underpinned by the concept of continued learning[59] – policies themselves can be thought of as experiments, which in the process of implementation produce evidence on how they are working.

We need to look beyond our current analytical techniques and incorporate broader approaches to understanding the promotion, protection and restoration of health. However, a useful first step would be to recognise the hegemony of current reductionist research frameworks which in many situations are inappropriate.

Conclusion

In recent years there has been a search for new policy instruments which reflects widespread dissatisfaction on the part of policy makers with established ways of providing health services. The current approach to NHS organisation has been called the third way in healthcare reform, a theoretical approach that emphasises a mixed economy utilising the dynamics of competition but with the public interest in mind. These reforms are symptomatic of a much broader agenda to modernise and improve public services as a whole.

This chapter has argued that there are limits to the ability to act rationally within the healthcare system and has called for a fourth way in healthcare which accommodates complexity insights. It recognises that complexity science is not a single theory but a 'meta-view', focusing on the patterns of relationships within organisations, how they are sustained, how they self-organise and how outcomes emerge. Within this framework there are a number of theories and concepts, many of which are contested. I have suggested a pragmatic approach, drawing on complexity metaphors when they seem to work in practice and are useful, and replacing them into the toolbox when they are not.

Complexity does not offer ready solutions to organisational change but shifts the gaze. It emphasises the limits to knowledge and predictability, and the importance of history. It changes the focus from outcomes to process and counsels that analytical and predictive power can only be gained by standing back, not by analysing a system in more detail. It emphasises network over hierarchy, the importance of trusting rather than checking and guards against reductionism. This does not obviate the need for the scientific method – both approaches are complementary. However, simple structures in healthcare organisations are rare and in many cases boundaries, relationships and attributions are uncertain.

Within the context of the NHS there are a number of obstacles to the development of the fourth way. These arise from the dissonance between the view of the world of policy makers and researchers who develop frameworks to direct and facilitate decisions in healthcare and the view of those who commission and provide it. Academics remain trapped in their paradigms as they seek to make reality fit their disciplinary matrices rather than the more logical converse. Funding spirals, and assessment exercises and internal politics often divorce them from service commitments.[60] Inevitably, the institutionalised theory that is created bears little relationship to the pragmatic requirements of end users. A first step would be for researches to work more closely with those they seek to influence.

At a government level, policy makers are unable to acknowledge publicly the limitations on their abilities to act rationally. The result – a gap between the expectation of government and the aspirations and capabilities of the health service. The political election cycle always favours quick fixes rather than programmes designed to bring about lasting change in NHS culture and the emphasis continues to be on deliverable targets that can be linked to government policies. Government remains a master institution. The simple rules remain unchanged – ministers decide/professionals deliver; politicians centralise credit/diffuse blame.

The move to a fourth way is also constrained by the history of the system. Organisations do not start with a clean slate from which ideal choices can be made. Systems develop within the framework that they have inherited, building on what has gone before. Often, organisations are memorials to old problems, institutional residues that reflect the historical processes through which problems have been tackled.[61] Policy change inevitably takes place against a background of limited room for manoeuvre. For example, extended lead times due to the long training requirements of health professionals limit flexibility in health service manpower development.

The essential first step to organisational change in the NHS is to shift the focus to a complexity frame of reference. Recognising the NHS as an emergent complex system and moving it towards a simple complex system is the next step. The emphasis moves to one of diversity and innovation, a complementarity of competition and cooperation and an emphasis on simple system goals within a culture of learning. The focus is on setting boundaries and removing obstacles to development and innovation. These developments require trust and the empowerment of individuals, but the NHS remains locked in many bureaucratic routines that still rely on control and distrust. Instead of searching for and trying to impose order, policy makers, researchers and practitioners must promote rich interaction, not to find the best way but to provide the healthcare system with a stable framework within which it can learn, adapt and innovate.

Over 60 years ago, the economist Keynes suggested that 'we need to invent wisdom for a new age and that in the meantime, we must appear unorthodox, troublesome and dangerous.'[62] Is complexity science this new wisdom – a meta-view that accommodates all aspects of organisational life that could offer genuine opportunities for cultural change and health service development? Or is it just a passing fad, articulating common sense and emphasising that we should all be nice to each other? Two features seem irrefutable. First the dominance of linear orthodoxy has been challenged. Second, genuine cultural change can only occur through the facilitation of a bottom-up organisational emergence rather than top-down systems engineering.

The science of complex adaptive systems may or may not be the new wisdom that Keynes calls for. But one thing is clear – his call to action is long overdue.

References

1   Black N (2001) Evidence based policy: proceed with care. *BMJ.* **323**: 275–9.

2   Sheldon T (2001) It ain't what you do but the way that you do it. *Journal of Health Services Research and Policy.* **6**: 3–5.

3   Holm S (1998) Goodbye to the simple solutions: the second phase of priority setting in health care. *BMJ.* **317**: 1000–2.

4   Kernick DP (1998) Has health economics lost its way? *BMJ.* **317**: 197–9.

5   MacKiver S, Baines D, Ham C *et al.* (2000) *Setting Priorities and Managing Demands on the NHS.* University of Birmingham, Health Services Management Centre, Birmingham.

6   Mannion R and Goddard M (2001) Impact of published clinical outcomes data: case study in a NHS hospital trust. *BMJ.* **323**: 260–3.

7   Marshall M (1999) Improving quality in general practice: qualitative case study of barriers faced by health authorities. *BMJ.* **319**: 164–7.

8   Thomas KJ, Nicholl JP and Coleman P (2001) Use and expenditure on complementary medicine in England: a population based survey. *Complementary Therapy Medicine.* **9**: 2–11.

9   Hayes B and Haines A (1998) Barriers and bridges to evidence based clinical practice. *BMJ.* **317**: 273–6.

10 Salisbury C, Bosanquet N, Wilkinson E *et al.* (1998) The implementation of evidence based medicine in general practice prescribing. *British Journal of General Practice.* **48**: 1849–51.

11 Lipsky M (1980) *Street Level Bureaucracy: dilemmas of the individual in public services.* Sage, New York.

12 Royston G (1998) Shifting the balance of healthcare into the 21st century. *European Journal of Operational Research.* **105**: 267–76.

13 Plsek P (2000) Re-designing healthcare with insights from the science of complex adaptive systems, crossing the quality chasm: a new health system for the 21st century. *National Acadamy of Sciences.* **322**: 355.

14 Iles V and Sutherland K (2001) *Managing Change in the NHS: a review for health care managers, professionals and researchers.* NCCSDO, London.

15 Ouchi W (1980) Markets, bureaucracies and clans. *Administrative Sciences Quarterly.* **25**: 129–41.

16 Harrison S (1988) *Managing the NHS: shifting the frontier?* Chapman and Hall, London.

17   DHSS (1983) *NHS Management Enquiry Report*. Department of Health and Social Security, London.

18   Department of Health (1989) *Working for Patients*. HMSO, London.

19   Le Grand J, Mays N and Mullingan J (1998) *Learning from the NHS Internal Market*. King's Fund, London.

20   Giddins A (1994) *Beyond Left and Right: the future of radical politics*. Cambridge Politics Press, Cambridge.

21   Department of Health (1997) *The New NHS: modern, dependable*. The Stationery Office, London.

22   Checkland P (1981) *Systems Thinking, Systems Practice*. Wiley, New York.

23   Greenberg D (1997) NIH resists research funding linked to patient load. *Lancet*. **349**: 1229.

24   Department of Health (1998) *The Health of the Nation: a policy assessed*. HMSO, London.

25   Smith R (2001) Why are doctors so unhappy? *BMJ*. **322**: 1073–4.

26   Stacey R (2001) *Complex Responsive Processes in Organisations*. Routledge, London.

27   Department of Health (1988) *A First Class Service: quality in the new NHS*. Department of Health, London.

28   Fraser S (2000) *Beyond Turf and Territory: leadership principles for unravelling the stranglehold of organisational boundaries*. Learning Through Partnership, Buckinghamshire.

29   Marshall G (1994) *Oxford Dictionary of Sociology*, Oxford University Press, Oxford.

30   Davies H and Mannion R (2000) Organisational culture and quality of healthcare. *Quality in Healthcare*. **9**: 111–19.

31   Maynard A (1996) Rationing healthcare. *BMJ*. **313**: 1499.

32   Cohen M, March J and Olsen J (1974) A garbage can model of organisational choice. *Administrative Science Quarterly*. **17**: 1–25.

33   Hogwood B and Gunn L (1984) *Policy Analysis for the Real World*. Oxford University Press, Oxford.

34   Miller W, Crabtree B, McDaniel R *et al.* (1998) Understanding change in primary care practice using complexity theory. *Journal of Family Practice*. **46**: 369–76.

35   Plsek P and Wilson T (2001) Complexity, leadership and management in health care organisations. *BMJ*. **323**: 746–9.

36 Zimmerman B and Plsek P (1998) *Edgewar: insight from complexity science for healthcare leaders.* Irving, VHA.

37 Garside P (1999) Learning organisations: a necessary setting for improving care. *Quality in Health Care.* **8**: 211.

38 Davies H and Nutley S (2000) Developing learning organisations in the NHS. *BMJ.* **320**: 998–1001.

39 Argyris C and Schön DA (1996) *Organizational Learning II.* Addison-Wesley, Reading, MA.

40 Brewick D (1998) Developing and testing changes in the delivery of care. *Annals of Internal Medicine.* **128**: 651–6.

41 Fraser S and Greenhalgh T (2001) Coping with complexity: educating for capability. *BMJ.* **323**: 799–803.

42 Puttman RD (2000) *Bowling Alone: the collapse and revival of American community.* Simon & Schuster, New York.

43 Welsh T and Pringle M (2001) Social capital – trusts need to recreate trust. *BMJ.* **323**: 177-8.

44 Fox A (1974) *Beyond Contract: work, power and trust relations.* Faber and Faber, London.

45 Berwick D (1997) Medical associations: guilds or leaders? *BMJ.* **314**: 1564–6.

46 Royston G and Dick P (1998) Healthcare ecology. *British Journal of Healthcare Management.* **4**: 238–41.

47 Foucault M (1991) Governmentality. In: G Burchell, C Gordon and P Miller (eds) *The Foucault Effect: studies in governmentality.* Harvester Wheatsheaf, London.

48 Light D (2001) Managed competition, governmental and institutional response in the UK. *Social Science and Medicine.* **52**: 1167–81.

49 Funtowicz S and Revetz J (1994) Emergent complex systems. *Futures.* **26**: 568–82.

50 Seedhouse D (1994) *Fortress NHS: the philosophical review of the National Health Service.* John Wiley, Chichester.

51 Kline R (2000) From evidence based medicine to evidence based policy. *Journal of Health Services Research and Policy.* **5**: 65–6.

52 Campbell M, Fitzpatrick R and Haines A (2000) A framework for design and evaluation of complex interventions to improve health. *BMJ.* **321**: 694–6.

53 Kernick D (2000) The impact of health economics on health care delivery. A view from primary care. *Pharmaco-economics.* **18**: 1–5.

54 WHO (1996) *European Healthcare Reforms: analysis and current strategies*. World Health Organization Regional Office for Europe, Copenhagen.

55 Honigsbaum F, Richards J and Lockett T (1995) *Priority Setting and Action: purchasing dilemmas*. Radcliffe Medical Press, Oxford.

56 Butler J (1999) *The Ethics of Healthcare Rationing: principles and practices*. Cassell, London.

57 Hunter D (1997) *Desperately Seeking Solutions*. Longman, London.

58 Kernick D (2000) Bridging the gap between theory and reality – a call for vernacular health economics. *British Journal of General Practice*. **50**: 684.

59 Walsworth-Bell A and Chang J (1999) *Promoting Research for Health Services*. Open University Press, Milton Keynes.

60 Kernick DP, Stead J and Dixon M (1999) Time to refocus the academic effort. *BMJ (Editorial)*. **319**: 206–7.

61 Pratt J, Gordon P and Plamping D (2000) *Working Whole Systems: putting theory into practice in organisations*. King's Fund, London.

62 Mannion R and Small N (1999) Postmodern health economics. *Health Care Analysis*. **8**: 255–72.

CHAPTER SEVEN

Clinical governance and complexity

Kieran Sweeney and Paul Cassidy

Summary

This chapter sets the history of clinical governance in the context of the 'new' NHS, and shows how the 'system' of implementation of clinical governance has several key features of complex adaptive systems. In particular, the rich interaction of the agents embedding clinical governance in a locality will produce self-organising behaviour (reflected in the plethora of different structures, committees, personnel and activities) which through time will locate the system of clinical governance around a particular attractor or pattern of behaviour, which in turn will co-create the emerging behaviour of the system. We speculate how the trajectory of a system of implementing clinical governance might move to a different attractor as a result of non-linear influences on the system, for example through the unexpected resignation of a clinical governance lead or a national requirement to make public the business of a primary care trust (PCT). Later in the chapter we turn to the mathematics of complexity to describe innovative mechanisms for assessing the degree to which any system – including a system of clinical governance – is integrated, that is how well connected its components are.

The aim of the chapter is threefold: to root the metaphors

and insights of complexity firmly in the clinical governance arena; to demonstrate the value of so doing; and to reflect on how specific techniques in the complexity of mathematics can help clarify the day-to-day work of assessing how well clinical governance has become embedded in any locality.

Introduction

The purpose of this chapter is to explore the notion of clinical governance from the perspective of complexity. How can the principles, metaphors and analyses developed under the broad umbrella of complexity help us understand clinical governance? How can complexity help us understand how clinical governance works, or how well it has been embedded by organisations?

After setting the historical scene, acknowledging the political origins of clinical governance, we will argue that the implementation of clinical governance constitutes a complex adaptive system, and can benefit from the insights of the complexity sciences. We will explore self-organisation and emergence as they relate to clinical governance; we will then speculate on the relevance of some of the conventions from the mathematics of complexity.

Background

In the UK NHS the ideas of clinical governance have become central to both the development and control of service provision. The origins of clinical governance are unmistakeably political. Quality and accountability form the central planks in a series of government documents which set out the Labour party's agenda for modernising the NHS.[1] Based on the 'third way', a compromise political strategy balancing the tensions between the traditional and modernising wings of the Labour party, the duty of quality was placed on all healthcare organisations.[2,3] This strategy was included in Section 18 of the Health Act 1999, which also made explicit commitments to building a health service that was responsive to the needs of patients, carers and the wider public. This was a sea change for the NHS. In addition to the conventional requirement for chief executives in health authorities or trusts to sign the annual financial report, guaranteeing probity in the handling of public money, there was now a new guarantee in relation to the quality of clinical care. In primary care, clinical governance was to be implemented by primary care groups (PCGs), which are now becoming PCTs – more autonomous bodies with extended commissioning responsibilities. Initially, 481 PCGs came into existence in April 1999, each serving populations of approximately 100 000. These groups had three broad responsibilities: to improve the health of the population, develop primary and community services locally, and commission some secondary care services. More than half had become PCTs by April 2002.

Clinical governance

Clinical governance has been defined as a system through which NHS organisations are responsible for continuously improving the quality of their services and safeguarding standards of care by creating an environment in which excellence flourishes.[4] The implementation of clinical governance requires the integration of seven key activities, shown in Box 7.1.[5] Clinical effectiveness, clinical audit and the use of clinical information are the three most familiar categories to practising clinicians. Risk management which includes error reporting and significant event auditing (SEA) is possibly the least well-developed activity, certainly in primary care. Continuing professional development, human resources and the patient experience complete the septet. None of these activities on their own constitute clinical governance: all are needed for a balanced policy. The trick is to integrate them all appropriately.

Box 7.1 Components of clinical governance

- Clinical effectiveness.
- Clinical audit.
- Use of clinical information.
- Risk management.
- Continuing personal and professional development (CPPD).
- Human resources.
- Patient experience.

This approach allows us to operationalise each of the components or themes of clinical governance as working principles, based on an understanding of the relevant literature and policy documents. In turn the working principles can be operationalised through specific activities which, if undertaken, constitute evidence that a particular pillar of clinical governance is being implemented. Table 7.1 illustrates this for risk management, showing the working principles on the left and the specific activities derived from these on the right.[1] This model will be referred to later in the chapter as it brings in the notion of connectedness, that is of integration between a principle, the strategy to implement it and specific operations which evidence its application.

Table 7.1 Turning risk management into practice: principles and activities[1]

Working principles	Specific activities
Learn from complaints and mistakes	Introduce a program of SEA meetings Assess how many practices are holding SEA meetings Develop a program for rolling out SEA to practices not holding such meetings
Regular review of practice systems	Direct evaluation of in-house practice complaints systems Collate evidence of how practices review and learn from complaints
Develop occupational health service (OHS)	Make a business case for OHS and secure funding Make the service available to all practices of the PCG/PCT Build in an evaluation of the service

The aim of a clinical governance programme is to ensure that all the components are well developed and appropriately implemented in everyday practice. Although there is no definitive method for implementing clinical governance, a number of models exist. For example, the Commission for Health Improvement (CHI), which has a statutory duty to assess the degree to which all NHS organisations have implemented clinical governance, has based its approach loosely on the Baldridge model (Figure 7.1). Here, the strategy and vision of an organisation, if properly defined, will lead to the appropriate use of resources and manpower in a way which will feed into and directly benefit an individual patient's experience. Again this model stresses the connection between the parts of the programme and their proper integration, a notion we will return to later in the chapter.

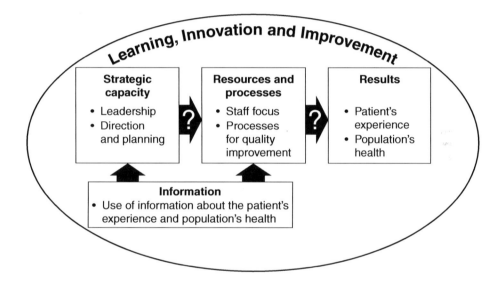

Figure 7.1 Baldridge Model. Adapted for Commission for Health Improvement reviews.

This chapter asks how the metaphors and analyses from complexity can help us to understand better the wide-ranging notion of clinical governance. The first step is to satisfy ourselves that clinical governance constitutes a complex system.

Clinical governance as a complex adaptive system

Table 7.2 shows, in the left-hand column, the features of a complex adaptive system. In the right-hand column are the corresponding attributes of clinical governance as it is embodied and implemented in primary care organisations.

Table 7.2 Complex systems and clinical governance

Characteristics of a complex system[4]	Corresponding features of a clinical governance programme
Complex systems have a large number of components.	Clinical governance is implemented by a large number of agents from a range of professions who try to integrate the seven key components. The agents can act at various levels of the system, from the centre (Department of Health) to region and then local level, right down to the individual practice level.
The interaction of the parts of the system is rich and diverse. Any element in the system can be influenced by and can influence many others. The interactions are non-linear.	Because a large number of elements are involved and an even larger number of agents of individuals are associated with the process of developing clinical governance, the interaction is rich and diverse. Within a clinical governance system small influences may have a large impact and vice versa. One example is the small report linking autism with the MMR vaccine which had a large impact on vaccination rates.[6]
Complex systems have a history which co-creates their present.	At the macro level, the history of clinical governance arises from political dissatisfaction with the historical development of the NHS.[1] At the local level, it will be implemented in localities in different ways depending on the local context and history.
Complex systems are capable of self-organisation under conditions far from equilibrium.	As PCGs developed, their structure was influenced and changed along with the local complexion of clinical governance; constituent practices all developed their own in-house structures and approaches to clinical governance.
Complex systems are open, they interact with their environment, and it is sometimes difficult to define their boundaries.	Clinical governance develops a quality in any locality which reflects the special characteristics of that group, their history, pressures, priorities and needs. This can change unexpectedly, e.g. in response to political changes in NHS policy, (e.g. mandatory data for NSFs). Issues of funding, relationships with social care, secular variations in health and alterations in the social context (housing, arrival of refugees, increased crime) all produce an unpredictable theatre in which clinical governance evolves.

We argue that Table 7.2 summarises the view that the activities which implement clinical governance have the characteristics of a complex adaptive system. The range of activities is diverse as is the nature of the professional groups involved in developing it. While doctors may dominate numerically, nurses, managers, social care professionals and citizens all have their role to play, and can influence the direction clinical governance takes. The nature of clinical governance will reflect the history, locality and community of the professionals who have the responsibility to implement it. This will give it a definite local quality.

The diversity of agents and their actions ensure that the connections between different parts of the system are rich, unpredictable and complex. But, more importantly, the interactions are non-linear, i.e. they cannot be predicted on a simple cause and effect model. For example, a relatively innocuous decision to stand down by a health professional responsible for clinical governance locally might have extremely serious repercussions for the PCG if there is no obvious or willing successor. In contrast, where a fairly major change, such as the move of a PCG to PCT status might alter some parts of the system (e.g. the medico-legal responsibilities of the Board), that change may have relatively little impact on other parts of the system, such as constituent practices, whose day-to-day activities might remain unaltered. The system is inherently unpredictable: unexpected changes and sudden deviations from tightly crafted plans are not just likely, but guaranteed. Witness the introduction of the National Service Frameworks, with mandatory data sets to be collected at PCG level, or the unexpected restructuring of health authorities in England, which destabilised the relationships between a PCG and its health authority.

Clinical governance and basic concepts of complex systems

Let's accept that the above analysis supports the view that clinical governance operates as a complex adaptive system. What are the basic concepts in complexity that might help us understand more clearly how clinical governance works or doesn't work in primary care? We propose two key ideas which provide helpful insights:

- self-organisation
- attractors.

Self-organisation

Self-organisation describes the ability of a system when far from equilibrium to produce fresh behaviour unpredictably, without a master plan. Although it was first described in relation to a chemical reaction (the so-called Belousov Zhabotinsky reaction), lots of complex adaptive systems exhibit this property.[7] Perhaps the most frequently quoted example is the 'boids', or the tendency of a collection of birds to fly in a flock formation.[8] On the face of it, this looks like pretty complicated behaviour, as the flock swirls and twists almost, it seems, with a life of its own. But flocking behaviour can be explained by three simple rules:

- maintain a minimum distance from the other birds
- match the velocity of the other boids in the neighbourhood
- try to move towards the perceived centre of the flock.

If you think about it, a bird flying in such a flock exhibits many of the behaviours of components of a complex system. There are no specific rules which dictate how and when a flock may form. Each bird is reacting to other components (i.e. the other birds) in the locality. No one bird is completely aware of what the whole flock is doing and no bird is in charge. The actions of individual birds influence the context in which the other birds are flying. The activity of flocking is truly an emergent behaviour of the interrelated actions of the component units of the system.

Such behaviour is not confined to animal activities like flocking. The stock market exhibited self-organising behaviour when it crashed temporarily worldwide after the bombing of the World Trade Centre and recovered about one month later. In this upheaval, the combined actions of the market's agents contributed to unpredictable emergent behaviour, namely a focused interest in the purchase of gold, antiques and rare furnishings. Many large commercial companies have altered their organisational behaviour in relation to an ever-changing hostile environment. Oticom, a Swedish manufacturer of hearing aids did just this. The staff eschewed their conventional offices and office furniture, and developed nomadic offices containing a mobile file cart, laptop and mobile phone. This flexibility allowed them to interact with whoever was most appropriate in their company with an ease that the constraints of the previous company structure had not permitted. Arriving at work one day, the managing director found that his mobile office had been wheeled into the marketing department as his colleagues felt he needed to spend more time there.[9] Here was self-organisation, with new patterns of behaviour emerging without a blueprint, in an organisation interacting with its external environment.

Attractors

Complexity recognises certain patterns of behaviour in adaptive systems which we referred to in Chapter 1 as attractors. The notion is helpful as it gives a broad, although relatively undetailed, picture of how a system is operating. Attractors can be seen in general practices. Some practices will exhibit patterns of professional excellence, for example with partners gaining Fellowship of the Royal College of General Practitioners by Assessment (FBA) or achieving external accolades such as Investors in People, or developing a quality assurance department in-house and educating nursing staff to specialist or practitioner status. In such practices clinical and professional excellence can be described as their attractor. The trajectory of the practice, that is the path which the practice as a 'system' will trace out through time, will stay close to the attractor notion of clinical excellence. Developments, innovations, new appointments or alterations to administration will tend, in such a practice, to reflect this notion. In colloquial terms, such an attractor is summed up as 'the way we work round here'. In contrast, other practices might build up large patient lists, run long surgeries, agree as a partnership not to have locum doctors, and cover each other for holidays. This kind of practice might have business or financial excellence as its attractor. Here, any proposed innovations will be evaluated (perhaps subconsciously) for their compatibility with the business excellence attractor. So, if such a practice were faced with the evidence that long appointments and smaller lists were good for patients, it would have great difficulty moving its trajectory (pattern of behaviour) away to trace out a new trajectory around the fresh attractor. This highlights the importance of trying to understand a practice's attractor when change is needed. Change is more easily adopted if it is compatible with the attractor state of an organisation. And what may seem initially like resistance to change may better be understood as the exhibition of an attractor state which is inconsistent with, but understandable in, the context of new circumstances. For example, there was considerable funding some years ago for mini-clinics for a range of conditions from asthma to overseas travel. A proportion of practices did not hold such clinics and resisted this change. Some of these did so because the innovation was not evidence based and there was no clear indication of how patients might benefit. For these practices, the innovation may have been considered incompatible with their existing attractor, clinical excellence.

We argue that healthcare organisations exhibit self-organisation and emergent behaviour as they implement clinical governance. Here are some examples to support our view.

When the person responsible for clinical governance realises the importance of, say, SEA, complexity allows them to consider how such a development might best be set up. They may set up a group of people to develop SEA, but the specific activities and interactions of the members will not be determined in advance. Over time, the way the group acts will co-create an emergent behaviour which will in turn influence the way in which the idea is developed on the ground; the group members need not be given a blue print or specific instructions about how to go about their task. Their attractor, that is the pattern of the combined actions, will be simply to enable all practices in their constituency to have been introduced to the idea of SEA by a specified time. When they approach practices, they may not have a uniform model, but try to tap into the practices' attractor states, recognising how the history, culture and particular team in the practice combine to produce their characteristic practice behaviour. So, some practices, who thrive on innovation (their attractor) will jump at the first short presentation on SEA.

Other practices, for example, may feel besieged by change and will need another approach. Maybe their attractor is excellent clinical care, and initially such a practice might see SEA as an impediment to getting on with the challenging task of delivering such high clinical care. An approach which taps into this attractor is more likely to succeed in nudging the system towards the new behaviour, than one which adopts a 'one size fits all' approach. For such a practice it might mean simply starting with short clinical meetings including, for example, an event where, despite the best of intentions, a patient experienced a medical emergency. Another group of practices, who feel that their community service is paramount (e.g. in a deprived area), might merit an approach focused on their attractor. Here, patient concerns relayed to the reception staff might be the entry route.

Complex responsive processes

In our explanation of the value of considering the concepts from the complexity sciences for clinical governance, our emphasis has been on the way individuals interact in the system. We stressed, for example, the importance of recognising mental models or what makes individual professionals 'tick' as described by David Kernick in Chapter 6 – from which will emerge, through the collective and interrelated actions of the team, a practice's attractor. Ralph Stacey, one of the UK's acknowledged experts in the implications of complexity science for organisations, has developed this idea of the quality of interaction between individuals by introducing the term *complex responsive processes* to underpin both the formative potential for these interactions, as well as describing how these interactions themselves are shaped by the emerging behaviours of the system: they construct the system's attractor, and in turn are co-created by that attractor – all in the absence of a blueprint.[10] This view has profound philosophical implications; it supports the proposition that the future is constantly being co-created in the present. This presents some theoretical problems for managers, who are charged with having responsibility, but whose system is being created and shaped by influences which they cannot fully control. The view also has profound implications for clinical governance. Clinical governance is not something which is delivered to a community of agents, but is rather constructed by them via spontaneous communications and non-linear interactions with the wider environment.

So, if we are trying to embed a system of clinical governance, a wise approach requires us to be aware of the mental models or the beliefs of the agents, to understand how the agents make connections (do they meet formally or informally, by e-mail or telephone) and develop some simple rules to guide the evolution of the relationships. In this way we can influence or at least understand the pattern of communication which determines which attractor the system settles around.

This has serious implications for predictability. Our model suggests that it is usually pointless to draw up a master plan, fleshed out in detail and delivered as a *fait accompli* to the community. There are times when a big idea will alter the trajectory of a system, bringing it to settle near a different attractor. For example, when it was decided that PCG board meetings were to take place in public, the system had to reorganise itself to distinguish between matters which could be circulated in public and those which could not, and to construct defensible criteria for distinguishing one from the other. For clinical governance, this model suggests that it may be better to stand back and observe the system responding to the 'new rules' introduced into the programme (like new ideas about clinical governance) and then facilitate the system to develop those ideas spontaneously.

Out goes the command and control approach. In comes the careful, thoughtful nurturing and building on what is already there (the principle of sensitivity to initial conditions which we identified as one of the features of complex systems). And gone is the certainty of success, always illusory even with command and control approaches. Sometimes the latter approach will be spot on, for example where there is a large amount of agreement about the nature of a system, and a similar degree of certainty about how the system will respond. Organising the flu vaccination campaign in a busy practice is an example of when the command and control system might be appropriate. At other times, where the nature and trajectory of the system is complex, several tacks may have to be taken. An example might be a practice which decides on a root and branch reorganisation of its practice nursing arrangements. When approaching change in complex systems, the only thing which remains certain is unpredictability.

Educating for clinical governance: the implications of complexity

If we agree that it is helpful to regard the implementation of clinical governance as the description and shaping of a complex adaptive system, with non-linearity and rich interaction as the key features, what educational methods are best suited for the task? Fraser and Greenhalgh,[11] in their excellent essay on this topic, emphasised the notion of *capability* over *competence*. Competence, they argue, refers to the conventional educational pursuit of acquiring knowledge, skills and attitude. However, capability implies that individuals can develop sustainable abilities which allow them to adapt to a changing environment, and react to unfamiliar situations. As an example to illustrate the distinction, consider a young doctor in general practice carrying out a diabetes review. The doctor will need the basic competencies to carry out the appropriate tasks and give evidence-based advice. These competencies might be enough to sustain the doctor through a completely routine check with a compliant and knowledgeable patient. But consider the consultation with a young insulin-dependant diabetic from an ethnic minority, who is smoking and drinking, has not yet fully accepted the diagnosis of diabetes, and whose diabetic control is chaotic. This provides a different scenario, requiring the ability to react to novelty and to work effectively in an unfamiliar environment. Education for capability is what is required here.

The educational methods which develop capability are novel, non-linear, participative and formative. Fraser and Greenhalgh advocate two types of educational approach:

- transformational
- relational learning.

In transformational learning, information about their own actions is fed back to learners, and they are asked to reflect on that feedback, shape their actions accordingly and repeat the process, constantly seeking the new feedback information which will guide the evolving actions.[12] Relational learning requires an individual to be able to link together disparate pieces of relevant knowledge in a way which helps them react to unfamiliar contexts. The capable management of ischaemic heart disease does not require simply a slavish adherence to a guideline. The capable physician will be able to relate knowledge of pathology with pharmacology, critical appraisal, use of guidelines, electronic data searching skills, behavioural science in relation to lifestyle and patient-centred consulting styles.

The educational processes which support the acquisition of such skills are inherently non-linear. Fraser and Greenhalgh suggest a range of educational activities:

- small group teaching, teambuilding and role play
- self-directed learning, including mentoring and peer-supported learning groups
- informal learning such as shadowing or teachback, where a newly skilled novice rapidly engages in teaching to share and enhance understanding.

These observations on the educational methods best suited to complexity have implications for embedding clinical governance. The process of implementing clinical governance is inherently educational, and forms part of continuing professional development. Fraser and Greenhalgh's review helps us select educational methods compatible with the task of educating our professionals to deal with the unexpected.

Clinical governance: looking at the big picture from the complexity sciences

So far in this chapter we have focused on the details of complex systems, considering their implications for clinical governance, and then reflecting on the skills needed to adapt to such unpredictable ever changing environments. In this last section, we want to take an overview of clinical governance from the perspective of complexity. How might the complexity metaphors help us understand how the big pieces of the system hold together? We know that the relationship between components of a system is vital to understanding that system. Can complexity tell us anything about how solidly the components of our clinical governance system relate to each other?

Here, we propose two useful analogies from the mathematics of complexity: the idea of interacting hierarchies from set theory, and some basic ideas in matrix algebra. Let us consider each of these in turn.

Set theory and the notion of hierarchies

The conventional model of clinical governance, used for example by the Clinical Governance Support Team, stresses the notion of seven pillars of clinical governance (Figure 7.2) which, suggested by the very name itself, are vertical structures running in parallel, supporting a supra-structure, which they call the patient–professional partnership.[2]

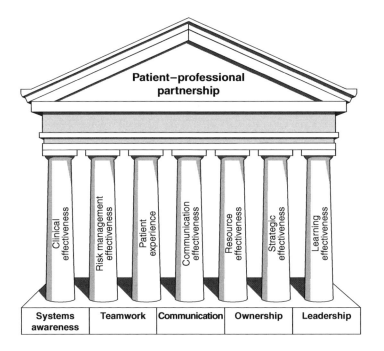

Figure 7.2 Vertical structure of pillars of clinical governance.

While this model helps us think clearly about each of the compo-nents of clinical governance, it doesn't tell us a lot about the way those components develop. The model is enacted by a variety of agents, who interact at all levels of the system, cross-fertilising ideas from one pillar to the other, each influencing, and being influenced by, the others in an iterative way. This is where the notion of interconnectedness helps. All the components are connected, and the agents implementing them are connected through their joint activities. Let us consider some theory from complexity which might help us think about these connections, and then refer to one interpretation of clinical governance which draws on it, albeit inadvertently.

Figure 7.3 shows a hierarchical diagram, which is intended to evoke the Russian doll model of connectedness, each subsection of the system fitting into, or being covered by, a corresponding piece higher up the system. The model derives from set theory in mathe-matics and reflects the almost universal feature of complex systems, namely that they tend to be organised in a hierarchical way with elements at the different levels interacting to produce complexity. In complex systems, complexity tends to increase as one moves up the system.

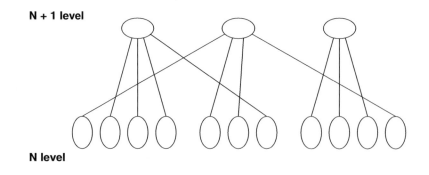

Figure 7.3 Set theory.

Suppose we have a set X containing a finite number of elements. Consider another set Y, whose elements are collections of elements of X. If all the elements of X are represented in the set Y, then Y is called a cover set for X. Y then exists at a higher level than X and, if we arbitrarily assign N as a level of X, then Y can be thought of as $N+1$. A simple analogy in healthcare would be an acute trust, as shown in Figure 7.4.

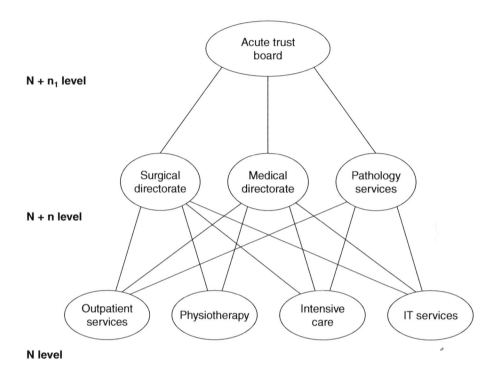

N + n₁ level

N + n level

N level

Figure 7.4 Set theory applied to healthcare organisations.

The model of clinical governance to which we referred earlier in the chapter alluded to this interconnectedness without explicitly using complexity vocabulary.[1] This model introduced the idea of the components of clinical governance, which are operationalised as *themes*, *working principles* (the mechanisms by which those themes are implemented) and *activities* (what actually happens to illustrate the implementation of the working principle). Table 7.3 shows the main themes of clinical governance and the working principles which implement them. Tables 7.1 (*see* page 126) and 7.4 below illustrate the specific activities which evidence the implementation of two of the working principles: risk management and the quality agenda.

Table 7.3 Themes of clinical governance and related working principles

Themes	Working principles
Collaboration	Health improvement programme Practical clinical governance meetings Develop relationships with social services
Risk avoidance	Learning from complaints Regular review of practice systems Develop OHS
Poor performance	Develop procedures for reporting concerns early SEA meetings Encourage nurse clinical supervision
Quality methods	Evidence-based practice Educational plans Develop audit programme
Culture	Citizen involvement Developing leadership Bottom-up change in thinking
Infrastructure	Secure proper funding Develop formal clinical governance teamwork and business meetings Work with IT department Develop good quality primary care clinical data

Reproduced with permission from Sweeney and Bradley (2001).[1]

Table 7.4 Quality methods: working principles and related activities

Working principle	Specific activity
Evidence-based practice	Encourage evidence-based practice in dementia service and develop protocol
Educational plans	Study days organised for all practices funded through PCG
Audit programme	Identify programme of audits which relate to the topics in the Health Improvement Plan (HImP), and arising out of SEA

Reproduced with permission from Sweeney and Bradley (2001).[1]

It is useful to think of the themes, principles and activities relating to each other like Russian dolls, sitting one within the other. In a nomenclature the specific activities would be the N level, the working principles $N+1$, and the theme $N+2$. For each of the themes a Russian doll set could be imagined, containing the principles within the theme and the activities within the principle. Each of the themes would then be described by a cover set and would in their turn be joined together in a larger cover set where the $N+3$ level would be the clinical governance strategy at board level.

We commend this model because it helps set out the connections between the components of clinical governance, the agents who embed it in a community, and the specific activities which evidence its implementation. It is a model which encourages the observer to stand back and see the overall picture. Using the model one can more easily explore for example how risk management fits in with professional development or how ideas from clinical effectiveness impact on other areas of clinical governance.

Clinical governance and Q connectedness

A second notion from the mathematics of complexity which might help us understand how the parts of a complex system such as clinical governance interrelate is drawn from matrix algebra, and the notion of simplexes. We freely admit to being novices in this area ourselves, but we argue that the thinking underpinning the mathematics is not only fairly straightforward but relates directly to events and connections which healthcare professionals meet every day. It is, in its simplest form, a numerical way of assessing how connected or integrated a whole system is. Let us take the mathematics a little further and then take a moment to underline its relevance to clinical governance.

The basic notion in this analysis regards the *structure* of any system as one component of that system's dynamics. The structure will consist of the interrelationship of the constituent elements, which is referred to as the system's connectivity. What this analysis tries to do is describe the degree of connectedness in any system in a precise mathematical, numerical way. The value of doing this is that it gives some indication of how well connected the components of the system are, which tells us something about how cohesive or integrated the system is. For clinical governance, we argue that this mathematical approach might be able to do the same, i.e. tell us how integrated a system of clinical governance is. Let us develop the mathematics, which is referred to as Q analysis,[13] a little further.

In any system, a simplex, i.e. a single component of a complex system, can be represented as a point, a straight line, a triangle, a tetrahedron or any higher dimensional polyhedron with an increasing number of sides. In mathematical conventions, the *dimension* of any simplex is equal to one less than the number of its vertices. That is, a point has zero dimension, a line one dimension, a triangle two dimensions, and a tetrahedron 3 dimensions, and so on. The dimension, as you see, indicates the nature of the space occupied by the simplex. A simplicial complex, then, is the association of individual simplices in a single system; the simplices need not actually share vertices, but can be connected by an intermediate chain of simplices. Figure 7.5 shows one such complex. Remember, that in representing a complex system like this, the analysis serves to emphasise the connections between the components. The formula uses the term 'Q connectedness' to describe the degree of relationship between two simplices in a complex. In the system shown in the diagram, simplex B and D are Q connected at level 1, as they share a straight line, the base of the two triangles, while simplex C and E are Q connected at the zero level, as they are connected only at a single point.

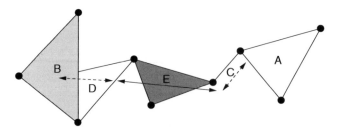

Figure 7.5 A simplicial complex.

These structural properties and their associated behaviour define the complex system, and the presence of connections between the components indicates a dependency between one component of the system and another. The precise number of parts in any system is not really important, as one can define the nature of a part, depending on the level of description in which one is interested. A system's complexity is a function of the interest of the observer.

These notions of *simplices* and their connectedness has led mathematicians to develop a formula for describing the eccentricity of a simplex within a complex, i.e. a numerical way of describing how integrated (or not) any part of a system (or simplex) is within the complex. The formula allows mathematicians to calculate whether a simplex is strongly or weakly integrated into a complex. Mathematicians do this using a matrix which represents the information stored in a simplicial diagram in numerical form, where the components are set out in horizontal and vertical lines. The matrix is a way of representing the pictorial structure set out in our example as a set of numbers. Let us consider an example from general practice looking at how information is disseminated to key subgroups of the practice's population. We accept straight away that the example serves simply to illustrate the potential in this technique: our matrix oversimplifies the way in which information actually flows in practice in order to demonstrate in principle how the connectedness of the agents in the system can be represented diagrammatically.

Consider as a 'system' the way in which information on evidence-based practice flows from professionals to the relevant patient group in a practice. One can imagine in this system, a relationship or set of connections between the professionals and the target group, where the relationship would exist if, and only if, that professional was actively involved in disseminating evidence-based advice to the target. One could imagine five sources set out as Y1 to Y5 below, and four target populations X1 to X4.

Y1	Midwife
Y2	Doctor
Y3	Health visitor
Y4	Practice manager
Y5	District nurse

X1	Expectant mother
X2	Children under 5 years
X3	Elderly patients
X4	Disabled patients

One could then draw up a matrix table in which the population of patients was linked to the source of information from the professional if, and only if, that professional could act as a resource for evidence-based practice for a member of that group. That would describe their connectedness within the system, and the greater the degree of that connectedness (which the mathematicians refer to as the Q connectedness), the stronger the integration of the components in the system. The matrix would look something like this, where 1 indicates that a relationship exists.

	Y1	Y2	Y3	Y4	Y5
X1	1	1	1	0	0
X2	0	1	1	0	0
X3	0	1	0	1	1
X4	0	1	0	1	0

One can then begin to see how these components are related in an imaginary simplicial complex, and begin to calculate how connected that complex is, using the notion of Q values. Using the top line to explain, there are three points of connection, so the Q value, i.e. the dimension of connectedness, is one less, namely 2. So is X3, which we could say was Q connected also at level 2. The other X components, X2 and X4 look as if they are more weakly Q connected. Thus for differing values of Q, the following statements could be made:

$$Q2 = X1, X3$$
$$Q1 = X1, X2, X3, X4$$
$$Q0 = X1, X2, X3, X4$$

It is possible to represent such a matrix pictorially as a simplicial complex. Figure 7.6 shows the simplicial complex of the matrix above. Presented in this way, this simplicial complex shows specifically that the system seems to be pivotal around component Y2, the doctor. It highlights a potential vulnerability in the system, if that component operates inappropriately or incorrectly. The general point about representing systems in this way is that one can begin to make observations about the degree to which the system is integrated.

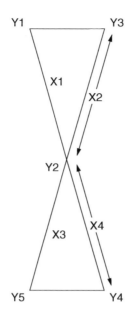

Figure 7.6 Simplicial complex drawn from matrix for information sharing.

Now, as we have depicted it, this system is oversimplified and its degree of integration can be assessed merely by glancing at the matrix. But in a system with 15–20 or more related components, some mathematical formula is going to be necessary to work out the degree of integration or eccentricity. Mathematicians have done just this, estimating the degree of integration of predators and prey in a forest, and perhaps even more strangely, the way in which certain scenes are integral to Shakespearean plays.[14] This explanation may begin to sound arcane, but we argue that the notion of simplicial complexes and their connectedness offers real possibilities for calculating the degree of integration in a system. For example, by representing in matrix form the components of clinical governance and the agents who implement it, and then converting that into a simplicial diagram, one could begin to make observations about the degree of integration or potential vulnerability of the clinical governance system.

We don't propose to take the mathematics further at this stage, but we suggest that further work on this notion could help us understand what the degree of integration of a system with a huge number of components, for example clinical governance system, is.

Those who want to take the mathematics further could dig deeper into Johnson's work on Q analysis.[15]

Conclusion

In this chapter we have argued that the implementation of clinical governance can usefully be understood as a complex adaptive system. This interpretation allows us to explain how the seemingly complex patterns of behaviour in such a system can be understood at the macro level, as the system's attractor. The model encourages us to focus on the interaction of the agents within the system, and we have given examples of how the agents can self-organise in reaction to new changes in the environment, without having to be given a blueprint for such novelty. We have introduced some basic ideas from set theory and connectedness to tempt us to examine how these approaches can help us understand the big picture, for example how the macro elements of clinical governance relate and integrate. Equipping ourselves to deal with this new explanatory model will require non-linear educational methods, and we have commended Fraser and Greenhalgh's essay on this topic. We argue that in reality, clinical governance is ever changing, its course unpredictable, and its direction always vulnerable to unexpected influences. A linear explanatory model, which tries to understand the system by reducing it to its components, and to control the system with the illusion of predictability will no longer do. Complexity offers us more productive insights.

Acknowledgements

We are very grateful to Frances Griffith for her helpful comments on the drafts of this chapter. We are indebted also to Dr Barry Tension for his invaluable help with the mathematics sections.

References

1   Sweeney K and Bradley N (2001) Clinical governance in primary care. In: J Secker-Walker and M Lugon (eds) *Advancing Clinical Governance*. Royal Society of Medicine, London, pp. 125–37.

2 Secretary of State for Health (1997) *The New NHS: modern, dependable*. The Stationery Office, London.

3 Ham C (1999) The third way in health care reform: does the emperor have any clothes? *Journal of Health Services Research and Policy*. 4: 168–73.

4 Scally G and Donaldson L (1998) Clinical governance and the drive for quality in the new NHS in England. *BMJ*. **317**: 61–3.

5 Donaldson LJ and Muir Gray LA (1998) Clinical governance: a duty of quality for health organisations. *Quality in Healthcare*. **7**: S37–44.

6 Petrovic M, Roberts R and Ramsay M (2001) Second dose of measles, mumps and rubella vaccine: questionnaire survey of health professionals. *BMJ*. **322**: 82–5.

7 Cohen I and Stewart J (1994) *The Collapse of Chaos*. Penguin, New York.

8 Kelly K (1994) *Out of Control: the new biology of machines*. Fourth Estate, London.

9 Pinchot G and Pinchot E (1996) *The Intelligent Organisation: engaging the talent and initiative of everyone in the workplace*. Berrett-Koehler, San Francisco, CA.

10 Stacey R (2000) *Complex Responsive Processes in Organisations*. Routledge, London.

11 Fraser SW and Greenhalgh T (2001) Coping with complexity: educating for capability. *BMJ*. **323**: 799–802.

12 Thorndike E (1992) *The Fundamentals of Learning*. Teachers College Press, New York.

13 Degtiarev K (2000) Systems analysis: mathematical modelling and approach to structural complexity measure using polyhedral dynamics approach. *Complexity International*. **7**: 1–22.

14 Casti J (1994) *Complexification: explaining a paradoxical world through the science of surprise*. HarperCollins, New York.

15 Johnson J (1991) The mathematics of complex systems. In: J Johnson and M Loomes (eds) *The Mathematical Revolution Inspired by Computing*. Oxford University Press, Oxford.

CHAPTER EIGHT

Complexity and primary healthcare research

Frances Griffiths

Summary

Written from the perspective of a general practitioner also engaged in sociology research, this chapter explores how complexity informs primary care research in terms of what research is done and how it is done. The chapter first explores research studying complex social systems, each system nested within another, for example the family nested within the community. It describes how research methods explore the interactions and feedback both within and between systems, take account of their history and environment, and analyse the data to draw out social theory. It suggests that this theory is our attempt to identify the emergent properties of the social system within which we as individuals are nested. The chapter then considers clinical research, particularly that used to identify the safety and effectiveness of interventions such as randomised controlled trials (RCTs). This research method is rooted in the understanding that individuals are complex systems in a complex world, and can be useful for some types of interventions, particularly drugs. However, the more complex the intervention, the more difficult it is to undertake an RCT and the more alternative research approaches are able to provide the evidence needed. Finally, the chapter suggests that research that is specifically general practice based increases our understanding of the craft of healing and our understanding of how this craft is best manifest at this time and place in our complex world.

Introduction

This chapter aims to explore how the ideas of complexity may enhance our research, and the understanding of research, that relates to primary care. This includes any research that relates to the provision of first-line health and social care. Such research would aim to increase knowledge and understanding so that service providers may then be able to improve the care of individuals. Primary care research is undertaken by a range of healthcare professionals and organisations, by academics from many different disciplines, and by voluntary organisations and consumers of health and social care.

Primary care research draws on a range of disciplines including clinical sciences, epidemiology, statistics, behavioural sciences (e.g. psychology) and social sciences (e.g. sociology). Important contributions come from other disciplines too, for example engineering, history and philosophy. The study of the arts also informs our understanding of the provision of health and social care. The aim of this chapter is to provide an introduction to how the ideas about complexity discussed in this book relate to primary care research. The chapter will focus on the forms of research undertaken by social and clinical scientists, with a brief mention of philosophy in the final section.

I am writing this chapter as a general practitioner working in primary care in the UK NHS, and as a researcher trained in the discipline of sociology. This is made explicit to highlight the interaction and feedback that occurs in our complex world. I bring a particular perspective to clinical care and research influenced by my background, experience and context. This is so for all clinicians and researchers although it is not always made explicit, as the idea of objectivity is still influential in medical research. By 'objectivity' I mean the idea that an observer can observe a phenomenon without influencing it in any way. Medical research has been slower than most other disciplines in acknowledging the impossibility of any absolute objectivity.

As I engage mostly in research that takes a social science approach to primary care, I will consider this first, using examples from my own research and that of my colleagues. As a GP I am a user of clinical research, so in the second part of the chapter I will consider this form of research with more of a user perspective. Finally, I will briefly consider philosophy in relation specifically to general practice research, although the ideas may be transferable to other generalist health and social care professions. Many of the ideas I discuss here are not new. Complexity seems to offer a framework for integrating many existing theoretical ideas. I have not spelt out the origins of these ideas but have taken a more pragmatic approach, starting with what we want to understand through our research. This probably reflects my background as a practising clinician but can be baffling to those from the social sciences where it is normal to develop an argument from a critique of existing theory.

Complexity and the social science approach

Primary care research taking a social science approach aims to understand social systems and their impact on health and social care. The social systems may be:

- organisations such as primary care within a locality or a mode of service delivery
- socially meaningful groups of people such as patients of a health service, families or local communities
- society more generally including its culture, information exchange including the media, industry and commerce, and government.

The social science approach tends to ask questions such as, 'what is happening here?' and 'why is it happening in this way?'. 'Why has a social group or organisation developed the way it has, how is it being changed or could be changed, and what is the role of individuals, policy and social movements?'. Some research asks more specific questions such as, 'what is the best way of delivering a particular healthcare service?'.

Individuals, organisations, social groups and society have characteristics of complex adaptive systems.[1] Analogies between human systems and computer simulated or biological complex adaptive systems are only partial. For example, as humans are self-conscious they can potentially decide how to behave in a way that is not only a response to their local environment but also a response to a wider or longer-term plan or vision. The extent and usefulness of the analogies have been and will continue to be debated. However, considering individuals and social systems as complex adaptive systems may increase our understanding of our research processes and results. Individuals and social systems can be conceptualised as systems nested within each other and inter-acting with each other. For example, the individual is nested within the family, which is nested within the community. This in turn is nested within the wider society of which part is the organisation of health and social care.[2] Of course the reality is not a stratified structure like a pile of soup bowls, as a system may occupy several layers at one point and not at others, but there is a general layered effect.

I will take an example of social science research and explore how it uses the ideas of complexity. The research I will discuss is an ongoing project, which is part of a research programme examining how health technologies are shaped by society and in turn shape society.* Health technologies in this sense include medical inter-ventions such as diagnostic processes, drugs or surgical procedures, and aids for daily life such as wheelchairs and service delivery systems. The research question recognises that there is interaction and feedback between technological innovation and wider society. The individuals involved in the interaction and feedback may include those developing and providing technology, those using the technology as healthcare consumers, those observing or commenting on the technology publicly, such as in the media or in government reports, and privately, such as with friends and collea-

---

*ESRC/MRC funded programme 'Innovative Health Technologies'. http://www.york. ac.uk/res/iht/

gues. Both the social nature of the health technology, including the priority given by society to technological intervention and its effect on social norms, and the actual use of the technology, are shaped by the interactions and feedback. Some of the interaction and feedback occurs within a system such as a community or a healthcare organisation. Other processes of interaction and feedback occur between such systems, for example policy decisions at national level will impact on local use of a technology and local demand for a technology will exert pressure on policy decisions. Such interaction and feedback are a key feature of complex adaptive systems. The concept of complex systems nested one within the other helps us analyse the interactions between the different levels, for example between national policy and individual care provision.

There are broadly two approaches to studying this type of research question, a fine grain approach and a more coarse grain approach. Along with colleagues, I am currently undertaking a more fine grain approach, looking at health technologies focused on women in midlife to understand how these technologies are shaped by, and in turn, shape society. The health technologies are hormone replacement therapy (HRT), bone densitometry and mammography. Our research includes interviews with women in midlife, interviews with health professionals involved in providing access to the technologies, and recordings of consultations between women and health professionals where these technologies are being discussed. The interview data will tell us how women and health professionals describe their approach to the health technologies, their decisions about the technologies and what has influenced these decisions, now and in the past, and their view of their interactions with other people in relation to the technologies. The consultation data will provide a record of some of the actual interactions that take place.

Our research aims to recruit women and health professionals from very diverse backgrounds and settings. This recognises the importance of history and context for individuals, organisations and society. A characteristic of complex adaptive systems is that they are influenced by their history and continue to develop over time. They are also interacting with their environment and adapting themselves as the environment changes. This includes the physical environment and also the social systems within which they are nested. For example, a doctor may have changed his or her approach to discussing menopausal symptoms presented as a problem by a patient as HRT has become more widely researched, more widely used and as social norms about how women present themselves and about using the therapy have changed.

The research interview data will of course not give us all the detail of the processes that the women and health professionals go through, but a representation of them. It would be impossible to capture every thought and action, if it were we would have reproduced the complex systems involved.[3] During an interview the interviewee describes their perceptions and analysis of the processes involved in making decisions about and using the technologies. Thus the women and health professionals have done the first stage of analysis in understanding what is happening and why, from their individual perspective. In recording a consultation between a woman and a health professional, we are recording an interaction which has history, context and many interacting influences for both participants. However, the consultation may be managed in a relatively standardised way reflecting the health professional's training and experience, and the woman's past experience of managing health encounters.

The data collection described uses a fine grain approach. However, the research question may also be explored through a more coarse grain approach. Rather than looking at the micro processes of interaction between individuals, the research may look at cultural, policy or organisational issues at a regional or national level. It may also look at more global issues influencing the use of the technologies. Such research may involve, for example, reading published literature on the development and use of the technologies, identifying arenas for debate such as correspondence columns, assessing the responses to the technology in the media and from self-help and voluntary organisations, and reading policy and guideline documents. Data would be mainly documents, key informant interviews and observation. In complexity terms this approach explores the environment of the system in which the health technology is provided. The micro processes for individual women and health professionals are nested within organisational policy and processes, and social and cultural processes. including the 'information society'. The 'micro' and 'macro' interact with each other and influence health technology provision and uptake.

Analysis of the data involves recognising patterns and categorising them. Biological studies are leading to an understanding of how the brain recognises patterns. It seems that recognition of patterns in the natural world, such as bees recognising where nectar can be found, is a key mental process for animals. Humans have extended this to include maps of spaces and ideas.[4] In analysing the data collected in the research described above, the research team looks for patterns. These may be common to many individuals or situations or may be only identified occasionally. The patterns will be categorised, for example patterns of interaction between individual's attitudes and the environment leading to use or non-use of the technologies, or patterns of interaction between cultural norms and organisational processes leading to use or non-use. The patterns and categories emerge from the interactions between the researchers and the data. Done well this interaction will be two-way, working from the data as well as working from the research team's existing ideas. A feature of complex systems is that the character of each system emerges from the interaction of the component parts.[5] I may be stretching the idea of emergence here as the data is not an active agent during the analysis process, although it is produced from the interaction of the interviewee and researcher.

How do we as researchers see more than the patterns we already know about? After all, research is intended to increase our understanding of the world. I don't think there is one answer to this. Traditionally researchers work from existing knowledge, as in published literature and existing theory. Researchers compare their analysis to existing understanding and try to challenge it. Working as an interdisciplinary team of researchers brings different perspectives to bear on the same data: this can lead to new understanding. In complexity terms the new understanding emerges from the interaction and feedback that takes place during the teamwork. The patterns, once identified, can be tested through returning to data collection after analysis, looking for both confirmation and challenges to the analysis. Although I have described a qualitative approach to data, quantitative approaches can also be used that involve identifying patterns and categorising them, and looking for new patterns. Qualitative data can be coded so it can be used, along with quantitative data. One computer analytical technique for this is cluster analysis. This may lead to the identification of unexpected clusters or patterns, or it may not.

Using the patterns emerging from the data the research team aims to formulate further social theory. The theory is an analysis at the level of society, based on the patterns emerging from the specific research data. The theory should be transferable to other people, other places, and for the research described, other technologies. Social theory is relatively simple. It is a means of identifying emergent properties of a social system. I will use an analogy to explain what I mean. A tree is a complex system. We understand a great deal about it through looking at the detail of its structure and function. However, if we write down all the detail, we do not then have a picture of a tree. For this we have to take a photograph, paint a picture or draw two straight lines for the trunk and some curly ones for the branches and leaves. As social beings we cannot stand totally outside our social systems (we can stand totally outside a tree) and in studying our social systems we are studying something at a higher level of analysis than ourselves: we are nested in social systems. Our attempt to describe the emergent properties of the social system is our social theory.

Our understanding of complexity teaches us not to use theory as predictive, even though it may indicate likely outcomes in similar situations. For example, from theory it may be possible to work out how policy and practice could be altered to direct developments in a desired way, but the only way to see if any changes have the effect hoped for, is to observe again.

Research on organisations may use both the fine grain and coarse grain approaches described above. For example, studying the introduction of a healthcare technology into a healthcare system may involve collecting data on the organisational policies and procedures, the processes of decision making and their implementation, and how individuals and groups within the organisation respond to the policy changes and decision making. This approach is sensitive to issues highlighted by ideas of complexity. It recognises that the change under study may be only one factor influencing the development of the organisation. The history and environment of the organisation will influence its development, as will individuals within the organisation through their interactions with others. The change for the organisation, in this example the

introduction of a new technology, may result in very little alteration in the organisation or it may precipitate a major upheaval.
Similar organisations may respond differently to the same change,
for example because of differences in their history and context or
because of individuals championing a cause in the organisation.
This idea of non-linearity, where an influence is modulated
through interactions, is a key feature of complex systems. The
research approach described above is known as a case study and is
a common methodology in organisational research. For example,
Meads *et al.*[6] undertook a study focusing particularly on the
relationships between people in primary healthcare. Similar studies
on the function of network forms of organisation, identifying the
nature of relationships between individuals that lead to success for
the organisation, have been reviewed to inform the development of
primary care research networks.[7] Research methods, including
experimental methods such as the RCT, are also used in organisational research. I will return to consider this approach later in the
chapter.

The social science approach to research aims to understand
social processes and in its research methods often takes account of
the complexity of society. As its research examines the processes in
society which are part of each individual's everyday experience,
when its results and theory are presented, it is recognisable, almost
familiar. Any new understanding may seem small. Perhaps this is
particularly so for those not following the development of social
theory but using the results for their application to a craft such as
general practice. For practitioners working within our complex
changing society and constantly adapting to it, it is easy to loose
the perspective of earlier times and generations.

Complexity and the clinical research approach

The experimental method, particularly the RCT, is considered the
gold standard for clinical research. Although other research
methods are used they are considered to produce less robust forms
of evidence. The issue about evidence and its value has received
much attention in clinical circles in the last decade, as the
evidence-based medicine movement has become influential. This
section will suggest how the ideas of complexity may contribute to

moving forward the debate on evidence and the development of research methods.

As a GP, I regularly encounter at least three types of research, clinical, public health based and sociological, all of which have different perspectives on the same issue. For example, clinical research accepts that HRT exists and that it is potentially useful for the relief of menopausal symptoms and for the prevention of osteoporosis and cardiovascular disease. Clinical research assesses the risks of taking HRT and whether it makes a difference to menopausal symptoms, rates of hip fracture or ischaemic heart disease in the current context. Public health research may seek answers to questions such as why women in western industrialised nations suffer from osteoporosis and cardiovascular disease. Sociological research complements these approaches, and may ask how a health technology such as HRT influences and is influenced by society, or how far menopausal symptoms are exacerbated by the society in which we live.

Clinical research uses methods that allow it to say something relatively generalisable about an intervention. For example, the long-term risks and benefits of HRT may be assessed through an RCT, as is currently underway in the UK.* The design of the trial will provide results that are likely to be applicable to many women in the UK, and perhaps parts of northern Europe, the US and other westernised, industrialised and affluent places. The generalisability depends on the design of the trial but is always limited to a context, both time and place, as well as the population to which it applies. This type of research can be very valuable for clinicians as it helps us to understand the likely effect of clinical interventions on individuals. The research method allows us to do this systematically, so we limit the harm we may otherwise cause before we realise something is not useful! The interventions most commonly tested in clinical trials are those developed from laboratory medical research and biotechnology. The intervention has been developed at a different level of analysis from the individual, for example from work on the cell or part of the cell. From this body of research, those undertaking the

---

*Women's International Study of long Duration Oestrogen after Menopause (WISDOM) funded by the Medical Research Council, the British Heart Foundation and the Department of Health for England, Northern Ireland, Scotland and Wales.

clinical trial have a good idea of the likely effect of the intervention. If individuals were complicated machines rather than complex adaptive systems, it would be possible to work out the effect of the intervention on the individual from the knowledge of, for example, the cell biology. The need for clinical trials is rooted in the understanding, whether conscious or not, that individuals are complex systems and that all the effects of an intervention cannot be predicted from understanding the system at a lower level of analysis.

When using an experimental method such as the RCT, the context is controlled as much as possible to allow the researcher to identify the effect of the intervention on the individual. The unit of analysis is the individual. Statistical methods put the individuals into groups for analysis but the groups are not meaningful in any other way. These methods consider the individual as complex systems only in as far as the research recognises the need for controlling for the interactions of the individual with their environment and with the research. As a clinician, I continue to want evidence on the safety and effectiveness of many interventions we use, and I think the RCT is our best available method, particularly when two interventions, for example two drug therapies, are being compared.

However, after the RCT comes the transfer of this knowledge to the ordinary clinical setting. This includes testing the transferability of the piece of knowledge gained from the RCT to individuals who would not have been included in the original trial. Some try to make the transfer of results to the ordinary clinical setting easier through the way they design the RCT. Testing the transferability is also undertaken in the process of reviewing evidence and guideline development. Many different pieces of research, in slightly different populations, are brought together to try to strengthen the transferability of the results. However, complexity theory suggests that outcomes for complex adaptive systems can only be observed, not predicted. Therefore to see whether the results of an RCT do apply in clinical practice, we need to observe what happens to the individuals using the intervention. This may be possible through studying existing variation in how doctors practice, using their routinely recorded clinical data, including clinical outcomes. Such a study would be observing the repeated 'therapeutic trials' that we undertake with individuals in clinical practice, including those who would not have been included in the RCT. GPs have been called experts in treating patients who do not fit the inclusion criteria for clinical trials.*

The ideas from complexity help in clarifying the limitations of RCTs. The trials may not give us a particular answer for treating a particular patient. However, they do indicate the likely boundaries of safety and effectiveness for each intervention. Doctors are under an obligation from society to minimise harm, so, for an intervention such as a new drug we need to know the incidence of side effects and the likely benefits in order to make a judgement as to whether to use it at all. The information from drug trials tells us whether we are acting in what is generally considered a zone of safety, even though the trial cannot tell us whether the drug is safe for the individual patient. The understanding of individuals as complex adaptive systems is key to understanding medical fallibility.[8] As doctors, we cannot predict what is going to happen to an individual patient, however much evidence we have from research.

In clinical practice, understanding the individual as a complex adaptive system may also help us understand why things do or don't work as we might expect them to from the results of research. For example, we may use a drug for a particular symptom but it doesn't work. This may be because of factors in the patient's history or current environment that modulate the pharmacological effect downwards, for example the negative interaction of stress and analgesia. We also see unexpected changes such as Mrs Smith described in Chapter 4 where she suddenly improved after taking an overdose, and as in cases of blood sugar levels of diabetic patients that suddenly go very high or low despite careful monitoring and adjustment of insulin, diet and exercise, as described in Chapter 3.

Our understanding of complex systems may also help with understanding which clinical trials need to be done, and which can be done. Criteria for need include the balancing of risk and benefit as discussed above. For example, when penicillin was first introduced, it so obviously saved lives that an RCT was unnecessary. However, where risk and benefit are more closely balanced, clinical trials are helpful.[9] Linked with this, but taking a slightly different perspective, is the control or lack of control that an indivi-

---

*Prof Chris van Weel, President of the European Society of General Practice/Family Medicine at the European General Practice Research Workshop, May 2000, Maastricht.

dual has over the intervention. For example, drugs are powerful interventions over which the patient has no control after taking the drug, so trials are important for establishing safety and effectiveness as the patient needs to know they are taking something generally considered safe before they take it. However, for other types of interventions, such as sessions with a physiotherapist for those with incontinence, the patient is involved and has some degree of control at every stage of the process. They can just stop doing what the physiotherapist asks them to do. For this type of intervention, a detailed descriptive study may provide as much information about harm and clinical effectiveness as a clinical trial. Thinking back to the idea of complex systems nested inside each other may help us to understand this difference. The drug intervention is acting on part of the physiology of the individual. The physiological system is itself a complex system nested within the individual. The intervention is therefore acting at a lower level in the hierarchy of nested systems than the individual. Of course, it is hoped that influencing the physiology will help the individual. The physiotherapy intervention is aimed at the individual; the individual has to decide to do the exercises suggested and then carry them out. In theory the patient is in control of the intervention.

Criteria for whether a clinical trial can be done would also include the degree of control an individual has over the intervention. The more directly involved the patient is in the intervention, the more sophisticated the design of the trial has to be to take account of the influence of the individual over the outcome. However, more fundamental to the choice of methodology is the simple versus complex nature of the intervention. An intervention such as a drug is not itself a complex system, whereas an intervention such as counselling involves a complex system, the individual counsellor. The components of a system for health service delivery, such as anthroposophic medical centres,* are

---

* Anthroposophic medicine is an 'holistic' approach to healthcare delivered by a number of health centres in the UK NHS. (For a recent review *see* Ritchie J, Wilkinson J, Gantley M *et al.* (2001) A model of integrated primary care. *Anthroposophic Medicine.* **January**. Department of General Practice and Primary Care, St Bartholomew's and the Royal London School of Medicine and Dentistry, Queen Mary's, University of London.) A conundrum for those delivering healthcare in recent years has been how to demonstrate that it works, the subject of a conference in the UK in 1999: *Evaluation of Complex Interventions: the case of anthroposophical medicine*, hosted by the authors of the report above.

complex organisations or systems. Although it is possible to successfully conduct RCTs of such interventions, I would suggest that it becomes more difficult, and so more expensive, the more complex the intervention. The Stacey diagram can help clarify the differences (*see* page 107). RCTs are useful for interventions that fall in the bottom left-hand corner of the Stacey diagram, where there is a fair amount of certainty about how the intervention relates to the outcome, and of agreement about what the outcomes are. For example, in a trial of a new drug for the treatment of type 2 diabetes, the researcher will know a great deal about how the drug affects the blood glucose-related physiology of humans and will use an outcome measure such as glycosylated haemoglobin. (This is a measure done on a blood sample, which indicates how well the blood glucose has been controlled.) Interventions such as counselling and anthroposophic medical centres are further up and to the right in that diagram, where there is less certainty about how outcomes relate to inputs. For example, anthroposophic medical care takes a different approach to mainstream UK medical care from the very start of the process of assessing the patient, through to treatments. There is interaction between the system and the patient throughout. It is not possible to trace particular inputs to particular outputs in the way it seems to be with the new diabetes drug. There is also less agreement about the outcome. For example, in counselling there may be very general agreement that the outcome is that the patient feels better in some way, but that raises many questions about what that means to different people in different situations. If a counsellor had been seeing Mrs Smith before her overdose (*see* page 66), the counselling may have been deemed a failure, although the outcome for Mrs Smith was very positive. As a health professional I also see people who apparently do not gain from counselling at the time, but later on they realise some benefit. The Stacey diagram helps our understanding by providing a map on which we can try to place the interventions we want to research. However, as with all maps it does not fully represent reality. For example, in our complex biological and social worlds the two axes don't ever meet, as there cannot be absolute certainty about outcome or about how input relates to outcome.

Other elements of complexity theory help us understand the difficulty of undertaking RCTs for complex interventions. The complex systems, such as the counsellor or the anthroposophic medical centre, will be influenced by their history and local envir-onment and will be adapting to changes in the environment and in response to interactions and feedback within the system. Thus, although the systems in different times or places may appear super-ficially similar, their development as complex adaptive systems may be very different. Therefore, their effect as an intervention on individuals may be different overall or their effect may appear similar overall, but may be very different for different individuals. However, it is possible to undertake trials of complex interventions, for example a trial of counselling in primary care.[10] Some trials set up as rigorous RCTs may produce a wealth of detailed description that is at least as informative as the measured outcomes. Complexity theory provides a framework for questioning whether an RCT is the appropriate way of testing the safety and effective-ness of an intervention. A descriptive study may provide under-standing sufficient for answering these questions for the current context in which the intervention is used. As complex adaptive systems themselves, the interventions will be changing over time so such studies will need to be repeated as the intervention evolves and as the context in which it is used changes.

General practice research

In the earlier sections of this chapter I discussed how research always relates to a particular time and place, sometimes asking questions about what is happening and why, and sometimes taking the context as it is and asking questions about safety or effectiveness. I also mentioned the research disciplines that tackle these types of research. As a GP I am left asking what specifically general practice research is, rather than what research of another discipline that relates to general practice is. This question may also apply to other generalist healthcare professionals who are not tied in their practice of medicine to a particular technology or narrow specialty.

The activity of trying to assist with healing, including trying to prevent or relieve suffering, are activities of general practice and other health professions that have been present down the ages and across cultures. These activities seem to be relatively non-context specific, although how they are undertaken may vary a great deal depending on time, place and person, as we should expect for complex adaptive systems. On the dimension of time for example, a doctor's and a patient's approach to healing in twenty-first century England may seem very different from that of eleventh century England. This is on the time dimension for society. For the individual, the approach taken at different stages of the life course may be very different. For a particular disease, healing may manifest itself very differently at different stages of disease progression, for example the transition from active treatment to palliative care in terminal illness. There may of course be other time dimensions such as that of a healthcare organisation. Healing varies between cultures, and within a culture it may vary between different social groups. It varies according to other aspects of context such as war or peace, prosperity or poverty. Healing also varies according to the perspective of the individual. For example, a terminally ill man may suffer more because of the loss of his parenting role than from the pain of his tumour, and so the attempt to relieve his suffering needs to be adapted to this perspective. For another individual this may not be an issue.[11] Although healing is manifest in many different ways, the idea of there being an activity of healing is very persistent throughout human society. In complexity terms the need for healing may be an emergent property of human society. But what has this to do with general practice research?

It has been suggested that for general practice, 'what we need is not better research data but better philosophy', and that 'within the co-operative human activity that is general medical practice ... (there is) an intuitive concept of what the goods internal to the practice are'.[12]

This seems to suggest that we need to rediscover or remember what we know about the healing craft of general practice that is not tied to a specific context. What makes us, as GPs, good at healing? What are the 'goods internal to the practice' that Toon speaks of? Asking this does not assume general practice has a monopoly on healing but that healing is the core task for general practice. This rediscovery can be both a philosophical and a practical exercise.[12] Equally important is for us to continually ask how this healing craft can be best carried out in our current context. For example, how does a particular health technology help or hinder in the healing task? How does national policy or a local pattern of service provision enable or disable the process of healing?[13] How should we respond to pressures from society such as the changing health concerns in the community or the impact of the Internet? How do we as individuals influence our healing role? How is society's concept of healing changing as society itself changes? Understanding the healing role needs to be at the core of general practice research. This will involve both research undertaken by general practice and the integration of the results of other relevant research from many disciplines. The aim should be a deep understanding of healing and of how it can be best carried out by us, at this time and place, in this complex world.

Acknowledgements

The ideas in this chapter have been developed through discussion with many colleagues but in particular with members of the Complexity in Primary Care Group* and with my co-researchers, Professor Eileen Green, Dr Gillian Bendelow, Dr Kathryn Blackett Milburn, Dr Mick Carpenter and Professor Geoff Meads. I am indebted to the co-editor of this book for his encouragement.

References

1 Byrne D (1998) *Complexity Theory and the Social Sciences: an introduction.* Routledge, London.

2 Harvey DL and Reed MH (1994) The evolution of dissipative social systems. *Journal of Social and Evolutionary Systems.* **17**: 371–411.

3 Cilliers P (1998) *Complexity and Postmodernism: understanding complex systems.* Routledge, London.

4 Stewart I and Cohen J (1997) *Figments of Reality.* Cambridge University Press, Cambridge.

5 Cohen J and Stewart I (1994) *The Collapse of Chaos.* Penguin, Harmondsworth.

---

* www.complexityprimarycare.org

6   Meads G, Killoran A, Ashcroft J and Cornish Y (1999) *Can Primary Care Organisations Improve Health as well as Deliver Effective Health Care? Mixing Oil and Water.* HEA Publications, London.

7   Fenton E, Harvey J, Griffiths F *et al.* (2001) Reflections from organisation science on the development and evaluation of primary health care research networks. *Family Practice.* **18**: 540–4.

8   Gorovitz S and MacIntyre A (1976) Toward a theory of medical fallibility. *The Journal of Medicine and Philosophy.* **1**: 51–71.

9   Charlton B (1993) Rival concepts of health: science and medicine. *Journal of the Balint Society.* **21**: 12–16.

10   Ward E, King M, Lloyd M *et al.* (2000) Randomised controlled trial of non-directive counselling, cognitive-behaviour therapy, and usual general practitioner care for patients with depression. I: Clinical effectiveness. *BMJ.* **321**: 1383–8.

11   Cassell E (1991) *The Nature of Suffering and the Goals of Medicine.* Oxford University Press, Oxford.

12   Toon PD (1994) *What is Good General Practice?* Occasional paper 65. Royal College of General Practitioners, London.

13   Willis J (2001) *Friends in Low Places.* Radcliffe Medical Press, Oxford.

CHAPTER NINE

Conclusion

Frances Griffiths

When you started to read this book you may have hoped it would introduce you to something completely new. Having read it, or some of it, you may be overwhelmed by the new ideas or be feeling the opposite, doubting there is anything new here. You may also hold both apparently contradictory views at the same time or move between these different views. For those of us trained in the 'science' of clinical professions, particularly in those professions such as medicine, where the positivist view of knowledge is powerful, getting to grips with the different ways of thinking about the world explored in this book can be a difficult task, but can dramatically open up windows of understanding on issues we have struggled with in the past. This has been the experience of many of the clinicians in the Complexity in Primary Care Group.*

However, as we have come to understand more about the ideas of complexity, we have realised there are many existing examples of activity in healthcare where the ideas from complexity are in action. This book has identified some of these and they may be familiar to readers working in healthcare. This may lead you to think there is nothing new here – well there is and there isn't. Complexity is the nature of the biological and

---

*See the Preface for information about the Complexity in Primary Care Group.

social world so we live with it all the time. When the complexity is pointed out to us it seems very familiar. However, what is new is being explicit about the theory of complexity and about our use of it in the provision of healthcare. Complexity theory gives a name and a theoretical framework to a great deal of work that has already been, or is being, undertaken. The work is already underway because as healthcare providers we are practical or crafts people.

Listening to BBC Radio 4's programme '*In Our Time*', I heard about the development of inorganic chemistry and the periodic table in the nineteenth century. I was struck by the similarity with where we are with complexity theory in healthcare now, at the beginning of the twenty-first century. For many centuries the alchemists had maintained that there were four elements – earth, air, fire and water – and worked with this theory in their experiments. Meanwhile, in everyday life many elements were recognised and used for their different properties, such as those of tin, copper or iron. Alchemy and everyday life didn't recognise each other. However, while working with the theory of the four elements, alchemists developed many of the processes basic to modern chemistry. The methods were developed before the theory of modern chemistry.

The alchemists were misled in the interpretation of their results by their theory. In the 1860s the periodic table was developed and established, classifying the elements according to their relative atomic masses. With this new theoretical framework, chemists used the processes, already well practised, to identify most of the elements over a short time period and fill in the periodic table. Complexity theory may be for healthcare what the periodic table was for chemistry. The theory of complexity is a meta theory. It provides a framework for fitting together other theories or ideas, many of which have been developed from studying or working in the real world of healthcare, just as the periodic table provided a framework for fitting together the elements already known and used in everyday life. Complexity theory may help us look again at research data and gain further understanding of results that were difficult to explain or were explained as error. It may also provide a framework within which we can more confidently use the many skills and processes we already know for providing, developing and researching healthcare, just as the periodic table enabled the alchemists' skills and processes to be used in the development of modern chemistry.

The chapters in this book provide examples of how complexity theory is increasing our understanding of existing theory, research data and skills in healthcare. From this we can draw confidence in our work to research, develop and provide healthcare. However, we need to remain critical of our use of the complexity theory framework. Rigorously examining our ideas and work can be difficult using a theoretical framework that so closely reflects our everyday life experience. We are no longer able to divide our thinking into everyday life mode and 'scientific' mode. This could be very exciting, opening up all sorts of possibilities but it may also make critical thinking more difficult. Interaction and feedback may be part of the answer, working as teams to develop our thinking and ideas, policies and plans. This seems to have already been recognised in many areas of healthcare where interdisciplinary groups have been set up for service delivery, development and research.

I shall draw out some examples from the chapters in this book of how complexity theory provides a theoretical framework for our current work and future developments.

Critical confidence in piecing together theory and ideas developed from studying and working in the real world of healthcare

The encounter between the patient and healthcare professional has been studied over many years. Chapter 4 outlined the theories and ideas developed in general practice based on studying what happens in the consultation in general practice. Many aspects of this work resonate with complexity theory, for example, the recognition of the interaction of physical, psychological and social factors for a patient, the importance of what happens over time, and the interaction and feedback occurring within the consultation. Complexity theory provides a theoretical framework that will enable further studies to develop. Having this framework is important as, until recently, these theories and ideas have struggled to find a place in the knowledge arena of medicine. They did not fit with the prevailing theoretical framework. However, in practice, the theories have been recognised and used; for example, in medical schools the departments of general practice usually provide training for medical students on communication skills.

The NHS has been developing and changing since its inception. Chapter 6 outlined some of these changes and the theoretical ideas underpinning them. It also indicated some of the ways in which the health service has functioned despite the prevailing theory or policy including 'muddling through', the 'shadow system' and informal networks. Chapter 6 outlined theory about organisations which takes account of feedback mechanisms and approaches to management that use feedback and positive reinforcement. These familiar ways of working, ideas and theories can now be pieced together under the umbrella of complexity theory. Healthcare managers can more confidently use what they have found works in practice, along with these other ideas and theories, in developing appropriate approaches to each issue.

Clinical governance (*see* Chapter 7) also draws on theory developed from the real world of education, quality improvement, guideline and organisational development. This work has demonstrated the effectiveness of feedback to health professionals on their activity in promoting change and the importance of quality initiatives or guidelines being adapted to each particular local context. Complexity theory provides an overarching framework for understanding why.

These are just some examples where studying the real world of healthcare has led to the development of ideas and theory for use by health professionals and managers. One of the difficulties for health professionals and managers has been the apparent contradiction between these ideas and theories and the dominant theoretical perspective in healthcare. This has led to heated debate and often misunderstandings, for example between the proponents of evidence-based medicine and healthcare practitioners where the application of the evidence can be difficult and the patient's history and context may be an overwhelming influence. The apparent contradictions have also led to uncomfortable working where pragmatic decisions are played down as 'muddling through' rather than being complimented as the best approach to an issue. Through the understanding provided by complexity theory these apparent contradictions can be more easily understood.

Critical reinterpretation of clinical and research data

Chapter 3 has described how blood glucose may be manifesting a 'chaotic' pattern in individuals living with insulin-dependent diabetes. This idea begins to explain the blood glucose measures that have been difficult to explain using the equilibrium model of diabetes and that have therefore either been ignored or attributed to a fault in the individual's management of their blood glucose. This new understanding of the clinical data could bring major changes to the approaches used by individuals living with diabetes and by their healthcare professionals. The clinical data has been there for as long as blood glucose monitoring has been possible; it is the interpretation that has changed with the development of a new theoretical framework. Similarly in epidemiology (*see* Chapter 5), data on the incidence of disease is now being examined from a different theoretical perspective, raising the possibility of different explanations for the changing patterns of disease.

The complexity framework opens up new understanding through the reinterpretation of clinical and research data. This may sometimes involve using innovative methods of data analysis, and sometimes involve using the new perspective with tried and tested methods. With the burgeoning of healthcare data captured on computer systems, and the ability of computers to analyse massive data sets, there may be many new opportunities to use routinely collected clinical and administrative data in research. This is an exciting possibility but our discussions in the Complexity in Primary Care Group on this issue suggests at least two warnings. First, there is a risk of taking a purely reductionist approach to a complex system. There may be much to gain from looking at the details of a complex system, but this has to be done remembering that a complex system cannot be fully understood through studying the component parts, even if the study includes examining some of the interaction and feedback. Second, a great deal is known about the nature of clinical data through work already undertaken using routine clinical data, such as the General Practice Weekly Returns Service run in the UK by the Birmingham Research Unit of the Royal College of General Practitioners.* Researchers have already developed an understanding of the limitations of routine clinical and administrative data. In our enthusiasm for a new approach we must not forget these limitations.

Critical confidence in our healthcare activity

The provision of healthcare draws on both science and art, but itself is a craft. Practitioners of the craft, whether policy makers, managers, nurses, doctors, or other health professionals are taking part in the activity of healthcare provision, adapting their skills and knowledge to the situation and to the individuals in need of their attention. Skilled practitioners have learned their craft through experience and from colleagues and patients as well as through formal learning. Practising such a craft involves close engagement with our complex world and so we are already familiar with many of the ideas discussed in this book. Complexity theory may give us more confidence in the knowledge we gain from our practice, and provide an alternative framework for thinking critically about our experiences. At the inception of the evidence-based medicine movement there was widespread criticism of knowledge gained from experience, from colleagues and from mentors, as this knowledge had not necessarily been rigorously tested through research. This criticism was of value in pointing out the importance of critical evaluation of all our healthcare activity, although the movement's enthusiasm for certain types of research perhaps led to misunderstanding about this message.

Complexity theory provides a framework for understanding the value of knowledge gained in a particular context with a particular patient, and the limitations of this knowledge. A key issue here is the robust yet unpredictable nature of complex systems. An experience with one patient in a particular context may be very similar to experiences with other patients, as robust complex systems,

---

* http://www.rcgp.org.uk/rcgp/research/research_units/index.asp#Birmingham

such as individual patients, tend to respond to health problems or interventions in a similar way. By observing and comparing the outcomes we can build up categories of likely responses. However, complex systems are also unpredictable and we need to be prepared for unexpected outcomes. Positive unexpected outcomes rarely cause difficulty, as everyone is pleased. Negative unexpected outcomes can be difficult to accept and raise questions as to why, and was someone at fault. There may have been a specific cause or failure, but complexity theory suggests that it may not be possible to identify a cause. Studying unexpected outcomes, both positive and negative, may increase understanding of the complex system but cannot be sure to prevent the unexpected from happening. The experience of those engaged in healthcare can be used in a critical way to develop new understanding and new ways of providing healthcare, in partnership with other types of research and development.

For those of us working in the health service, complexity theory demonstrates how the day-to-day, local activity of providing healthcare is key not only to the immediate provision of services but to how those services develop, respond and change over time. We may work in a system designed at a different time and in a different place, but by working in the system we are changing and developing it. Complexity theory provides a framework for critically examining our health service processes. For example, is there sufficient feedback for the system to adapt and evolve? It can also reassure those who struggle to apply 'best evidence' or work with linear guidelines to know that the struggle can be understood and that it may be the nature of the evidence or guideline and not necessarily a personal failing that makes it difficult.

In the healthcare research arena, complexity theory can provide a framework for critically using the many well-developed and carefully refined research methods we already use as well as opening up potential for new methods. Interaction between researchers from different disciplines, and interaction with patients and carers as expert advisors, can lead to increased understanding of the many and varied perspectives on a health issue and lead to new understanding. In particular, this interaction will enable the development of analysis which takes account of the interaction between the different complex systems which have an impact on health, from national policy, through the local community and healthcare provision, to an individual's physiology.

Understanding healthcare activities in terms of complexity theory highlights the intimate link between healthcare, health service delivery, service development and research. Research is the critical eye that can be focused on any part of the healthcare system: policy through to physiology. It can look in detail at part of a system, take a step back and see the system as a whole or focus in and out through different systems. It can intervene in a system from outside or it can step into a system and observe from inside. Through observation, assessment and analysis, research can increase our understanding of our complex systems, and be immediately relevant to the development of the system if integrated into it. For example, healthcare professionals can use the critical eye of research on their own experiences, and those of their patients and colleagues, to increase understanding of a health issue. A manager can observe, assess and analyse organisational processes, put in place changes that may improve effectiveness of the organisation and observe, assess and analyse again. However, this is not an easy task and requires transparency and rigor in the research process. Perhaps more difficult is demonstrating the value of such research in a knowledge environment that considers the experimental method to be the best form of research. Complexity theory provides a framework for demonstrating the value of the many and varied methods of research we use and for moving towards greater integration of research, service development, service delivery and healthcare.

The way forward

This book aims to provide an introduction to complexity theory for healthcare. The authors and editors do not claim to have all the answers. Far from it, we offer this as a framework in need of refining and filling out. In 1869 the periodic table was described by Mendeleyev, and was based on the atomic weight of the elements. A later refinement was to use atomic number rather than weight, which removed certain anomalies. Many chemists were then involved in identifying the elements to fill out the periodic table. Similarly, complexity theory seems to provide a framework into which fit many ideas and observations. It may well need refining, as the periodic table needed refining, and it certainly needs filling out and testing for where and how the theory is useful in understanding our world. We invite you to help refine complexity theory and test it in your own healthcare arena.

Index

Page numbers in *italics* refer to boxes, figures and tables.